Transformough
Reflective Practice

Transforming Nursing Through Reflective Practice

Second Edition

Edited by
Christopher Johns
Dawn Freshwater

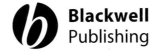

Blackwell
Publishing

© 1998, 2005 by Blackwell Publishing Ltd
Editorial offices:
Blackwell Publishing Ltd, 9600 Garsington Road, Oxford OX4 2DQ, UK
 Tel: +44 (0)1865 776868
Blackwell Publishing Inc., 350 Main Street, Malden, MA 02148-5020, USA
 Tel: +1 781 388 8250
Blackwell Publishing Asia Pty Ltd, 550 Swanston Street, Carlton, Victoria 3053, Australia
 Tel: +61 (0)3 8359 1011

First edition published 1998 by Blackwell Science Ltd
Second edition published 2005 by Blackwell Publishing Ltd

Library of Congress Cataloging-in-Publication Data

Transforming nursing through reflective practice / edited by Christopher Johns and
Dawn Freshwater.–2nd ed.
    p. ; cm.
  Includes bibliographical references and index.
  ISBN-13: 978-1-4051-1457-8 (pbk. : alk. paper)
  ISBN-10: 1-4051-1457-6 (pbk. : alk. paper)
  1. Nursing–Philosophy.   2. Reflection (Philosophy).   3. Self-knowledge, Theory of.
  [DNLM: 1. Nursing.   WY 16 T772 2005]   I. Johns, Christopher.   II. Freshwater, Dawn.

RT84.5.T73 2005
610.73–dc22
2004025007

A catalogue record for this title is available from the British Library

Set in 10/12.5pt Palatino
by Graphicraft Limited, Hong Kong
Printed and bound in India
by Gopsons Papers Ltd, Noida

The publisher's policy is to use permanent paper from mills that operate a sustainable
forestry policy, and which has been manufactured from pulp processed using acid-free
and elementary chlorine-free practices. Furthermore, the publisher ensures that the text
paper and cover board used have met acceptable environmental accreditation standards.

Visit our website:www.blackwellnursing.com

Contents

Foreword

A Meta-reflection on Reflective Practice and Where it Leads

Jean Watson

This revised edition of the work by Johns and Freshwater brings forth some of the futuristic views and evolved developments in the scholarship of reflective practice, combined with the most contemporary thoughts regarding philosophically guided reflection. If reflective practice is, at its most basic core, about 'seeing' and uncovering nursing at its core, then one of the rhetorical questions for scholarly discourse is how, where and what is the next level of exploratory depth for reflective practice? In other words, where would the work take us, if we allowed the work itself to philosophically and operationally inform us as a practice guide to the future? Could it be that this next turn takes us to an unexpected place, beyond the current generation of the work?

A meta-reflective lens: from–towards

As I allow the work to guide me, I see the next level of archaeological depth as a turn *from* reflective practice *towards* contemplative practice/to mindful practice/to conscious–intentional caring–healing practice for self. This next turn of the work goes beyond the early origins and careful, thoughtful, scholarly work to date, but allows the true practitioner of this field to go to a new place. For me, the work speaks in such a way that I am led away from a purely intellectual-knowledge focus *about* reflective practice, *towards* a wisdom path of personally *living* reflective practice. The question then is: how do I become the reflective practitioner in my day-to-day life? How does the work itself inform and guide my (and others') professional work and world?

To follow this phase to its core, the wisdom quest becomes a heart-centred quest, allowing for expansiveness and deepening of the work. Therefore, in this evolving wisdom quest the heart gets to inform the head, rather than the other way around. The wisdom, heart-centred focus towards authentically *living* reflective practice opens us up to our own personal world and we come face to face with our own individual practices.

Therefore, in this emerging model we are invited, personally and professionally, to engage in our inner and outer work, exploring our inner journey, towards the deeper level of the work. It is through such inner work that we are more able to witness the process and contribute to a transformation of the outer work.

If we follow this path and take it seriously to the next phase of depth to which it is leading, we enter a new space. In this next space we now have to pay close attention to our inner and outer personal development, our ontological competencies (Watson 1999) and to the very nature of the consciousness we are cultivating, whereas, in the past, we have paid much more attention to our technological, outer competencies for professional development and improving practice. Therefore, we now shift our focus *from* the professional practice of reflective practice, *towards* the more contemplative/intentional consciousness-cultivating practices of mindfulness of the nurse, him/herself. This *towards*-movement is a movement of heart-centred-wisdom practices.

As the work itself guides this future direction, this heart-centred personal wisdom practice uncovers the individual and collective values, ethics and professional commitments. They in turn sustain and expand the disciplinary and professional development of nursing and its science of caring.

If we consider a deep level of reflection, which transcends the obvious, we can seek wisdom-beyond-knowing; we tap into a level of reflection that asks moral questions and the broader question of why do we care for the other person (Norvedt 2003, p. 223). It is here that we share our connectedness and common bond of humanity, whereby one person's level of humanity reflects back on the other. Thus, one person's suffering is everyone's suffering. It is here in this deeper level of reflecting-upon-reflecting that we find a juxtaposition and intersection between the abstract–theoretical and the pre-reflective, ethical sensitivity in living out our day-to-day personal practice experience.

This ethical wisdom-beyond-knowing place evokes heart-centred practice; it becomes ontologically-based; it is informed by the very being, the very presence, and the compassionate awareness/awakening of the nurse in a given moment. The awareness shifts the discourse from an abstract/*professional*/ theoretical focus on reflective practice to a more contemplative, *personally ontologically cultivated* focus for a meaningful *living out of reflective practice*.

This expanded direction for following reflective practice into the future intersects with notions of transpersonal and ontological competencies (Watson 1999). That is, it takes us, individually and collectively, as practitioners and as a profession, beyond the ego-mind-centred, outer-chaotic world of practice, reorienting us towards working from the inside out. It is here we discover experientially the human-to-human connection that unites us for shared caring and healing needs across time and space. Thus, we can explore reflective practice within the context of what might be thought of as an ethical sensitivity of heart-centred wisdom practices.

Such a practice is referred to in wisdom traditions as the practice of *mindfulness*, in the sense of being aware, awake, conscious and intentional with one's presence and being in the moment; attending to the interplay between one's pre-reflective inner being and outer responses in a caring moment. It is when one is in this place of personal wisdom, gaining new and deeper insights, that a caring moment becomes more possible (Watson 1999). This movement towards a more contemplative/mindful practice opens up nursing to a field of what might be called *mindful caring–healing practice*.

A personal practice of mindful practice takes me and us beyond the current phase of thinking, well beyond the mechanics of care, and the conventional levels of discourse about practice as seen from an external lens. Sitzman (2002) frames a contemplative mindful-practice-view around Thich Naht Hanh's concept of *interbeing*. Zen master Thich Naht Hanh, in exploring interbeing, created the term to describe the intersecting and merging ideas of all levels of existence. That is, everything is interdependent and interconnected. By considering interbeing within a transformed reflective practice context, we again see that these practices and approaches take us to a different level of knowing-beyond-knowing, related to wisdom traditions and perennial philosophies. Such an approach to reflection is grounded in writings and practices of sages across time.

Thus, the cultivation of such work is to become more skilful in integrating the inner and outer, shifting one's lens from the outside to inside, from outer world to inner world. This shift moves from the professional–academic discourse, to a personal inner–outer dialogue to uncover pre-reflective wisdom and ontological–ethical compassionate caring competencies. The question now becomes how do we allow/enable the beauty that we are, to become the beauty that we do? How do we cultivate this reflective awareness/reawakening for beautiful, good, compassionate, caring practice? As noted earlier (Watson 1999, 2002b; Sitzman 2002) this deepening knowing-beyond-knowing comes from opening ourselves to heart-centred practices.

Heart-opening practices include a journey towards connecting matter with spirit, beyond ego self. They include personal commitments and practices such as formal meditation, prayer, breathwork, yoga, connections with nature, music, poetry, journaling, centring and other such forms of daily contemplation. This personal commitment becomes seminal to the personal authenticity of reflective practice and is the path towards more fully actualising nursing's authentic caring–healing work. This reflective practice of *being the beauty that we are* becomes the highest ethical and aesthetic contribution to healing. The height of human artistry is radiating one's inner beauty and light, through one's very being, mirroring and honouring the inner beauty of other human beings and all living things.

This form of commitment and authentic personal practice 'becomes a process of creating a spirit-filled sacredness and reverence around our work' (Watson 2002b, p. 6). With attention to the personal, ontologically evolved, pre-reflective nurse, we acknowledge we are working with our own and another's life force, energy-spirit and inner radiance and beauty that unite us in this shared human dilemma.

Caritas nursing: becoming *the caring field*

To engage in such a deep level of reflective practice requires the personal and daily practice of the nurse to undertake this commitment for ontological development of self. As the nurse does so, he or she *becomes the field of caring* in the moment. In *'being-the-field'*, so to speak, the nurse is part of transforming the larger system and even society, towards a higher/deeper level of moral evolution. This new field of practice for nurses who become the field might be called *'caritas nursing'* (Watson 2002a, 2004). It is the highest ethical commitment nurses can make to self and humanity itself. It is here where the wisdom of reflective moral knowing combines with one's inner energy and the radiance of love, beauty, compassion and human presence. The nurse who becomes-the-field is alchemically integrating the inner-wisdom, reflective, ontological insights and skill with technical knowledge, transforming chaotic practices into caritas nursing, whereby humanity and caring–healing are sustained.

This proposed direction for reflective practice is ancient and noble work that the nurse performs for self and other, helping to usher in a new era in human health and history. In revisioning reflective practice and allowing it to take us to its next evolution, we can posit nursing's ultimate contribution to society: *becoming the caring field*, thus, co-creating a moral community for true healing, offering a subtle, yet tangible, kind of world service towards an evolved humanity.

References

Norvedt, P. (2003) Subjectivity and vulnerability: reflections on the foundation of ethical sensibility. *Nursing Philosophy*, **4**: 222–30.

Sitzman, K. (2002) Interbeing and mindfulness: a bridge to understanding Jean Watson's theory of human caring. *Nursing Education Perspectives*, **23**(3): 118–23.

Watson, J. (1999) *Postmodern Nursing and Beyond*. Harcourt Brace, New York.

Watson, J. (2002a) website: www.uchsc.edu/nursing/caring.

Watson, J. (2002b) Intentionality and caring–healing consciousness: a practice of transpersonal nursing. *Holistic Nursing Practice*, **16**(4): 1–8.

Watson, J. (2004) *Communitas and Caritas*. Paper presented at 26th Annual Research Conference of the International Association for Human Caring, Montreal, 3–6 June 2004.

List of Contributors

Dawn Freshwater PhD, BA (Hons), RGN, RNT, FRCN
Professor of Mental Health and Primary Care at Bournemouth University, UK, and Foundation Chair in Regional Professional Studies, Edith Cowan University, Western Australia

Eleanor Gully RCompN, MA (Applied) Nursing, Cert. Counselling, CAT, HT, Cert. Reflexology
Formerly Nursing Lecturer. Practitioner/Therapist at Sophia Centre, New Zealand

Helen Hardy RGN, BA (Hons)
Head of Recruitment and Retention, North Central London Strategic Health Authority, UK

Amanda Howarth MSc, RGN
Clinical Lecturer in Health Sciences at School of Nursing, University of Sheffield, UK, and a doctoral candidate

Susan James PhD
Director of Midwifery Education Programme/Programme de formation des Sages-femmes at Laurentian University, Sudbury, Ontario, Canada

Louise Jarrett BA (Hons), DipHS, RGN
Clinical Nurse Specialist, Spasticity Management, National Hospital for Neurology and Neurosurgery, University College London Hospitals, UK

Christopher Johns RN, PhD
Reader in Advanced Nursing Practice, Faculty of Health and Social Sciences, University of Luton, UK

Ruth Morgan RGN, RM, DN, BA
Clinical leader in palliative care and a modern matron at a community hospital within Hertfordshire, UK

Bernie Pauly MN, BSc N
PhD candidate in nursing and research associate with the Ethics of Practice Research Team at the University of Victoria, Canada

Gary Rolfe PhD, MA, BSc, RMN
Professor of Nursing at the School of Health Sciences, University of Wales, Swansea, UK

Gillian Todd RMN, Diploma Nursing Care of the Mentally Ill in the Community, BA (Hons), Postgraduate Diploma Cognitive Therapy, UKCP (BABCP), Accredited Cognitive Behaviour Therapist
NHS Research Fellow in the Department of Developmental Psychiatry at Cambridge University, UK, working towards a PhD

Liz Walsh MSc, RGN
Commenced a PhD in prison health in 2003 and is currently working as a research fellow in prison health at Bournemouth University, UK

Jean Watson PhD, RN, HNC, FAAN
Distinguished Professor of Nursing and Murchinson-Scoville Chair in Caring Science at the University of Colorado Health Sciences Center, Denver, Colorado, USA

Chapter 1

Expanding the Gates of Perception

Christopher Johns

Aldous Huxley (1959) reflected on his experience of taking mescalin and its impact in enabling him to access the greater 'mind at large' and in doing so to circumvent the brain and nervous system as some sort of reducing valve. In other words, taking mescalin blew fuses and opened Huxley's mind to perceive things in new and different ways. Hence the title of his book, *The Doors of Perception*. As we go about our everyday business we take the world largely for granted and respond habitually. Meaning is projected into events that enable us to take things in our stride, and in doing so, reinforce our sense of self. Thus the multiple doors of possibility are not always visible: instead, existing knowledge and experience are defended as if the ego itself is threatened. The more we know, the more threatened we become when that knowing is challenged. A certain degree of anxiety and fear is useful for learning (see Joyce 1984; Casement 1985; Freshwater 2000). However, too much fear and anxiety is not conducive to learning. Perhaps we all need mescalin in the morning to heighten our perceptions, to lower our defences and open ourselves to possibility.

From a Buddhist perspective we are caught in a world of *samsara*, depicted by the cock, the snake and the pig – craving, aversion and delusion respectively – who chase one another around and around, locked into a world of greed, hate and ignorance. It is a restless world of seeking pleasure to avoid pain: what Freshwater (2003) refers to as 'toxic speed sickness'. We cling to what we know, for the small pleasures that we have, lest we lose even them. Yet, as Huxley (1959, p. 55) notes: 'the urge to transcend self-conscious selfhood is, as I have said, a principal appetite of the soul'. This message is reinforced by transpersonal philosophers such as Ken Wilber (1996) who makes a compelling argument that the goal of human evolution is to transcend self through increasingly higher levels of consciousness. Margaret Newman (1994), drawing on diverse theorists such as Young (1976) and Prigogine (1980), suggests that the role of nursing is to guide people (requiring health care) to grow through the health–illness experience towards higher levels of consciousness. She uses examples of people experiencing life-threatening illness and its impact in finding new, more positive meaning to life. In order for nurses to assist others through the process of expanding consciousness, they too need to be aware of their own need to work at differing levels of consciousness. Buddhists have struggled with such questions for a lifetime. The Buddhist path, it is argued, is a way to free self and others from this endless suffering and misery in order to realise our human potential and destiny. Perhaps mescalin can bypass the effort required to break free of conditioned existence but it is yet another form of avoidance, it is addictive, its effects are short-lived and, of course, it is illegal. So much for mescalin! Nevertheless, Huxley's message is clear: there is a mind at large that few of us rarely tap into that opens up possibilities for human growth. And herein lies the further *potential* of reflection. This potential is highlighted because I suspect that is not people's general perception of reflection. The aim here is to open the doors of your perception to reflection and its possibilities. If you want to slam the door shut on all this heady nonsense, ask yourself why. But in doing so, consider the words of Beckett (1969, p. 169):

> To be capable of helping others to become all they are capable of becoming we must first fulfil that commitment to ourselves.

I have always been drawn to Beckett's words simply because they offer a profound challenge to each of us who purport to care. The fulfilment of this responsibility must be the hallmark of professional practice. However, this is not necessarily easy work. Many nursing authors have taken up Beckett's challenge, turning the reflective gaze inwards towards self-transformation, self-care and self-reflection. Nevertheless, there continues to be a struggle against reflective practice, amid the belief that it is self-indulgent, narcissistic and selfish. This tells us something not only about the culture and context, but also about the way in which we relate to the self and to the ego (which tends to get a raw deal).

Describing (defining) reflection

The reflective traveller is faced with an array of definitions and models as possible guides. I have been developing my own description of reflection over many years. As a reflective practitioner, I constantly seek better forms of representation in light of new experience and insights. Hence description is preferable to definition, because definition implies an authority that I feel would be misplaced with regard to the idea of reflection.

> Reflection is being mindful of self, either within or after experience, as if a window through which the practitioner can view and focus self within the context of a particular experience, in order to confront, understand and move toward resolving contradiction between one's vision and actual practice. Through the conflict of contradiction, the commitment to realise one's vision, and understanding why things are as they are, the practitioner can gain new insights into self and be empowered to respond more congruently in future situations within a reflexive spiral towards developing practical wisdom and realising one's vision as a lived reality. The practitioner may require guidance to overcome resistance or to be empowered to act on understanding.

(Johns 2004a, p. 3)

From this description, reflection is both subjective and particular. It is a fusion of sensing, perceiving, intuiting and thinking related to a specific experience in order to develop insights into self and practice. It is vision-driven, concerned with taking action towards knowing and realising desirable practice. In doing so, it intends to resolve contradiction so that people can lead more meaningful lives. In other words reflection is purposeful.

Attempts, including my own, to 'know' reflection are essentially an intellectual effort to grasp something as if it had some sort of objective reality: a point of reference so that everyone would know exactly what it was. Such is the Newtonian nature of science: to know and control things. Perhaps as a technique reflection can be known, although the plethora of definitions and models indicates little intellectual consensus. Indeed, the diversity of opinions suggests that intellectual effort to know reflection is subjective. Reflection cannot be grasped because reflection *is* essentially a way of being in the world that is intuitive and holistic. Hence, by its very nature, it cannot be reduced into a neat conceptual analysis.

The practitioner reading this description of reflection, or in fact any other definition of reflection, is faced with interpreting the words into action. Put another way, how do you 'do' reflection? In response, theorists have constructed elaborate models to guide the practitioner into the mystery of doing reflection. Indeed I have contributed to this field with my own Model for Structured Reflection (MSR) that I constructed and have constantly tested and refined (Box 1.1). The ways of knowing shown against each cue in Box 1.1

Box 1.1   Model for structured reflection – 14th edition (Johns 2004a)

Reflective cue	Way of knowing
• Bring the mind home	
• Focus on a description of an experience that seems significant in some way	Aesthetics
• What particular issues seem significant enough to demand attention?	Aesthetics
• How were others feeling and what made them feel that way?	Aesthetics
• How was I feeling and what made me feel that way?	Personal
• What was I trying to achieve, and did I respond effectively?	Aesthetics
• What were the consequences of my actions on the patient, others and myself?	Aesthetics
• What factors influenced the way I was feeling, thinking or responding?	Personal
• What knowledge informed or might have informed me?	Empirics
• To what extent did I act for the best and in tune with my values?	Ethics
• How does this situation connect with previous experiences?	Reflexivity
• How might I respond more effectively given this situation again?	Reflexivity
• What would be the consequences of alternative actions for the patient, others and myself?	Reflexivity
• How do I NOW feel about this experience?	Reflexivity
• Am I more able to support myself and others as a consequence?	Reflexivity
• Am I more able to realise desirable practice monitored using appropriate frameworks such as framing perspectives, Carper's fundamental ways of knowing, other maps?	Reflexivity

refer to the way in which the cue tunes the practitioner into specific ways of knowing as delineated by Barbara Carper (1978):

- empirical – extant knowledge that provides the empirical basis for effective practice
- ethical – an appreciation of how best to respond in terms of societal benefit, expectations and norms
- personal – those things embodied within the practitioner that influence the way he or she sees and responds to the world
- aesthetic – the practical know-how and professional artistry used by each practitioner as they go about their work.

In accommodating these ways of knowing in the MSR, I identified a further domain which I termed 'reflexivity' (Johns 1995) to emphasise the impact of past experience on the present: the present turning back on itself to reflect on the way it has evolved from past experience. Such knowledge reflects the contextual – how knowing has been shaped by historical and contextual forces (see also White 1995; Freshwater & Rolfe 2001; Rolfe *et al.* 2001).

Carper's ways of knowing are a valid scheme for framing learning through reflection, although this scheme has tended to be too abstract for practitioners to interpret. Carper's scheme becomes practical when configured around aesthetic knowing (Box 1.2). So when practitioners describe a particular situation, they reveal their aesthetic knowing: the pattern for making sense of the situation, using clinical judgement and responding appropriately so as to realise a particular outcome, at least as they interpret it. The practitioner is then challenged to reflect on the way the empirical, personal, ethical and reflexive ways of knowing informed or might have informed their aesthetic response. A pattern of knowing emerges within the whole that can be appreciated and re-patterned towards realising more desirable practice in future similar experiences within a reflexive learning spiral for realising desirable practice.

I have explored models of reflection elsewhere (Johns 2004a) alongside other commentators (for example, Rolfe *et al.* 2001; Fitzgerald 2002). Sensible practitioners use these models creatively to help them see and learn through experience. A recent paper by Mary Woods (2003, p. 865), a lymphoedema clinic consultant who used the 1995 version of the MSR to reflect on her work with Kathryn, illustrates this. Mary writes:

> Reflection is an active process (Conway 1996) that enables healthcare professionals to gain a deeper understanding of their experiences with patients. Johns (1995) suggests that action may then be taken towards increasing effectiveness in practice. Learning through reflection therefore enables the healthcare professional to respond to new situations from a changed perspective. It links past experiences to personal, moral, political and social concepts that have had an influence on the individuals involved in each encounter. Subsequent reflection on these influences acts as a vehicle for action and change.
>
> Models or frameworks of reflection help healthcare professionals reflect on their practice effectively. They help to guide thoughts and focus attention on relevant

Box 1.2 Carper's fundamental ways of knowing (Carper 1978; Johns 1995, 2004a)

issues within the encounter. Johns' (1995) model for structured reflection adopts a humanistic approach, viewing the professional and patient as equal partners in creating the environment. The model uses simple questions that encourage a concern for the other person and is particularly fitting when reflecting on the interpersonal relationship between the professional and patient.

Mary chose the MSR because she felt it was in tune with her values and not merely an abstract technique. Jill Souter (2003) adapted the same version of the MSR to pay attention more explicitly to 'spiritual knowing' in palliative care. Although the use of the now outdated MSR is questionable, it does, however, seem to enable Jill to align herself with her practice values.

The risk with models of reflection is that they impose a (representation of) reality on the practitioner that forces a fit into the model rather than using the model as a creative opportunity: 'Our models are a prison. They are a way to explore self. They act as filters that accept what we believe and reject what seems otherwise' (Levine 1986, p. 53). The practitioner needs to see models for what they are, a sense-making tool rather than a thought prison (Johns 2002, p. 45).

If reflection is a path towards transformation, then practitioners will need to walk the path well. Linear models of reflection may be helpful to guide the novice reflective practitioner to take their first steps along the reflective pathway. Yet, even as they stumble in their efforts to walk, reliance on their chosen models needs to be confronted with encouragement to give way to their intuitive instincts. Models are no more than an *aide mémoire*.

Towards a more balanced perception of reflection

In a recent paper (Johns 2004b) I set out a typology of reflection spanning from reflection-on-experience to mindful practice (Box 1.3). In this typology

Box 1.3   The span of reflective practice (Johns 2004a, b)

Layers of reflection	Key theorists	
Reflection-on-experience Reflecting on a situation or experience after the event with the intention of drawing insights that may inform my future practice in positive ways.	Mezirow (1981), Schön (1983, 1987), Boyd & Fales (1983), Boud *et al.* (1985), Johns (2004a)	Doing reflection
Reflection-in-action Pausing within a particular situation or experience in order to make sense and reframe the situation so as to be able to proceed towards desired outcomes.	Schon (1983, 1987), Freshwater & Rolfe (2001)	
The internal supervisor Dialoguing with self whilst in conversation with another in order to make sense.	Casement (1985), Rolfe *et al.* (2001)	
Reflection-within-the-moment Being aware of the way I am thinking, feeling and responding within the unfolding moment and dialoguing with self to ensure I am interpreting and responding congruently to whatever is unfolding. It is having some space in your mind to change your ideas rather than being fixed on certain ideas.	Johns (2004a)	
Mindful practice Being aware of self within the unfolding moment with the intention of realising desirable practice (however 'desirable' is known).	Freshwater (2002), Johns (2004a)	Reflection as a way of being

reflection-on-experience is typified as a cognitive approach to reflection, that is, as something someone does. In contrast, mindful practice most typifies reflection as a way of being: a way that honours the intuitive and holistic nature of experience.

In my opinion, definitions of reflection as *reflection-on-experience* or *reflection-in-action* tend to reveal a (Western) cognitive approach that seeks to reduce experience into a rational understanding: a standing back from the situation to take an 'objective' view. Whilst this approach is useful it doesn't emphasise a view of reflection as a mindful, holistic and intuitive lens to view self within the unfolding moment. As Benner *et al.* (1996) assert, mindful practice is the essence of expert clinical judgement. It is the exquisite ability to appreciate the pattern of the unfolding situation from a position of deep ethical engagement within the situation.

Mindful practice

My quest for a more adequate representation of reflection led me to explore more diverse influences, most significantly Buddhist and Native American philosophy, that offered holistic and intuitive perspectives and balanced the cognitive approach. As with all things in life, balance is crucial for harmony. Whilst reason and rationality are important qualities, so too are perception, feelings and the senses if creativity is to flourish. This can be observed in, for example, the Taoist principles of yin and yang, the masculine and feminine, and negative and positive loops.

The Buddhist perspective would view reflection as a way to nurture and realise wise and compassionate practice within a strong ethic of doing good in the world. This understanding has strongly influenced my own work as a palliative care practitioner and complementary therapist towards easing suffering and nurturing growth by cultivating wise and compassionate care through reflective/mindful practice (Johns 2004c). Consider the following description of *bimadisiwin*:

> *Bimadisiwin* is a conscious decision to become. It is time to think about what you want to be. The dance cannot be danced until you envision the dance, rehearse its movements and understand your part. It is demanding for every step needs an effort in becoming one with the vision. It takes discipline, hard work and time. Decide to be an active participant in your life journey. It is rewarding. Embrace the joy your vision brings you, it is yours to hold forever. It is freeing, for it frees the spirit. It releases you to become as you believe you must.
> Believe in the vision of you
> Practice the vision
> Become the vision

(Jones & Jones 1996, p. 47)

In my view, this absolutely captures the spirit of reflection – this notion of knowing and realising vision as a way of being. Ask yourself: 'What do I aim to achieve at work?' 'What is caring?' 'Do I care?' 'Do I *really* care?' 'What constrains my caring?' Profound questions indeed.

Using descriptions of reflection like *bimadisiwin* opens the doors of perception as to what reflection is and helps confront my own constraints. I ask myself why I feel uncomfortable talking about Buddhism and Native American folklore with my students. Do I intuitively know they will label it flaky, hippy-dippy stuff and reject it? Are we so caught up in the technological world that such ideas are inherently threatening and must be resisted? If so, reflection will never realise its transformative potential. The MSR already incorporates Buddhist influence with the first cue 'bring the mind home' adopted from Sogyal Rinpoche's book *The Tibetan Book of Living and Dying* (Sogyal 1992).

Reflection is a path of self-awareness to become more self-conscious in terms of the actions we take towards realising our values or vision. Yet, as Young's theory of evolutionary consciousness (cited in Newman 1994) indicates, the decisions we make and actions we would take are constrained by our conditioning. As such we have to first unlearn or unwrap ourselves from these constraints, as difficult as that is because these constraints are deeply embodied and reinforced within the everyday world. It is as if we know our place within society and understand that to act out of place invites sanction from those more powerful keepers of tradition. Usually we self-regulate ourselves because we fear the consequences of acting out of place.

Milton Mayeroff (1971) writes about 'being in-place': the place a person needs to be in order to realise their values truly. So for myself, as a palliative care practitioner and complementary therapist, I need to be in-place to realise my vision of easing suffering and nurturing the growth of the other through their health–illness experience. Mayeroff contrasted 'being in-place' with 'knowing your place', a place determined by authority, embodiment and tradition rather than by values and a sense of autonomy, and which is often the wrong place to be if desirable practice is to be realised. Reflection then helps the practitioner to feel this tension between 'being in-place' and 'knowing your place' and the choices he or she needs to make in order to be in-place.

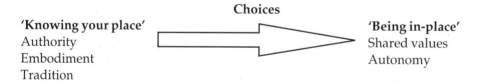

	Choices	
'Knowing your place'		**'Being in-place'**
Authority		Shared values
Embodiment		Autonomy
Tradition		

The reflective effort is to appreciate those forces that keep the practitioner in their place and constrain the necessary choices to move and be in-place; forces grounded in issues of tradition, authority and embodiment that limit the practitioner's ability to act autonomously on the grounds of rationality (Fay 1987). It is difficult to see beyond the normal self and the way one habitually thinks, feels and responds to the world. People are normative and take self for granted, often despite a deep gnawing of anxiety that indicates life is not satisfactory. Coming to realise that self leads a contradictory life and that one is not as competent as one believed oneself to be may throw people into an existential crisis and may lower self-esteem, at least initially. Feeling impotent to change the way self is or to confront the constraints that impede the realisation of one's values may be very frustrating and anxiety provoking, especially if the person perceives self as powerless.

Hence, reflection always requires guidance to challenge and support the practitioner along the reflective journey; challenge to surface, confront and appreciate the contradictions between one's reality and the realising of one's vision; and support to give courage to make the right choices and take steps to shift the conditions that constrain and to move into the right place.

Reflection as humanities

"Reflection opens the door of perception to reveal experience. This can be presented as a story, either spoken or written. It might begin: Many new names greeted me on the whiteboard that informed the bed location of each patient. A small red candle burns on the desk to honour a patient who had died in the early hours of the morning. A nurse turns to her colleague and says, 'We need to clean the Rose Room now the undertakers have taken the body.' The Rose Room is where people in transit to the undertakers are discreetly placed. 'Rose' softens the impression of a mortuary. The use of the word 'body' confirms the person's transition from life to death. This is normal hospice talk yet I feel a tinge of regret as I would prefer to hear the nurses talk of Violet or Mrs Morrison.

I visit Martha. She is asleep. Outside the room, Millicent, Martha's daughter, chats with nurses. Eye contact, a smile, as I leave the room. Shortly afterwards I bump into Millicent in the small kitchen.

I say, 'You're Martha's daughter?'

'Yes, I'm Millie.'

I inform her I am the complementary therapist and had popped in to ask Martha if she would like any therapy. Millie exclaims tearfully that she is unable to touch her mum, that she is frightened of the consequences. She feels guilty. I instinctively touch her shoulder as if to reassure her that it was OK to hold such feelings whilst simultaneously reading the signs to check out if my touch response was appropriate. She visibly relaxes. I acknowledge how tough it is to dwell with people, even our mothers, as they die.

Martha is awake. I kneel by her side. She gazes at me with slightly hostile eyes as if I represent a threat. She has refused all treatment and wishes to die now. She has a urinary tract infection (UTI) but has refused antibiotics. I inform her I am a complementary therapist but she mishears: 'I don't want physiotherapy.' I gently reiterate that I am a complementary therapist. Less threatened, she asks what I do. In response she says she was a healer and practised Reiki. She asks me to see her later after she has spoken with her daughter. In the meantime she agrees to an aroma-stone – I use sandalwood and lavender to combat the UTI odour, to help with the infection and to ease the anxiety in the room. Martha smiles as I leave her, as if we have a connection through our healing."

Reflection

Consider this text using the MSR cues (Box 1.1). In particular note the cue, 'To what extent did I act for the best and in tune with my values?' How would you determine the 'best' in this situation? Did I respect the daughter's and mother's autonomy? Did my actions benefit both daughter and mother? Did my touch violate the daughter's personal space and cause her some harm, especially as she has difficulty with touching her mother? Consider the cue 'What knowledge informed or might have informed me?' This is such a vast question in light of the extant knowledge available to me. Does such knowledge help me make sense of the daughter's response and despair and the mother's wish to die? Was my reassuring action in touching Millicent's shoulder appropriate in light of current research? Were sandalwood and lavender the best essential oils to help? Consider the cue 'What factors influenced the way I was feeling, thinking or responding'? Again a vast question to consider but at its core this question asks me how well I know myself and whether I am in the right place to realise desirable practice. These three specific cues illuminate the vast scope of reflection. Each of these cues can be addressed superficially, like scratching the surface of something very deep. Yet each cue, when listened to intently, takes me deeper and deeper into my experience as if carefully lifting back layer upon layer of veil to reveal the heart of self in the context of caring practice.

The experience with Millicent and Martha whilst apparently mundane on the surface is astonishingly profound. It is mundane in the sense that such experiences are commonplace within the hospice, and profound because of the intense feelings of the moment as someone draws close to death. Reflection always lifts experience out of the mundane into the profound: a sacred moment of dwelling with this woman and her daughter at such a moment in their lives. Reflection fosters a more sensitive and mindful approach to practice as I become more conscious and responsible for the decisions I make and the actions I take.

Instead of writing the story I could have painted the experience or written a poem. Art form seems to tap the right side of the brain where qualities of perception, imagination and creativity often lie dormant. Yet it is these very qualities that help to reveal the mystery of experience. As it was I didn't paint or write a poem in relation to my experience with Martha and Millicent, although my story telling has become increasingly poetic and less prosaic over time.

It is probably true to say that most of us lead habitual lives whereby much of experience drifts by with minimal attention as to the nature of the experience. Perhaps when the smooth flow of experience breaks down in some way, we pay attention to try to fix the breakdown and move on. Reflection offers a way of paying attention, of opening the doors of perception. We may thus become mindful of each unfolding experience in such a way as to enable us to learn from that experience and move towards realising more desirable and satisfactory lives. In doing so, we can become more effective practitioners: wiser, more perceptive, more compassionate and more skilful.

References

Beckett, T. (1969) A candidate's reflections on the supervisory process. *Contemporary Psychoanalysis*, **5**: 169–79.

Benner, P., Tanner, C. and Chesla, C. (1996) *Expertise in Nursing Practice: Clinical Judgement, and Ethics*. Springer, New York.

Boud, D., Keogh, R. and Walker, D. (1985) Promoting reflection in learning: a model. In *Reflection: Turning Experience into Learning* (Boud, D., Keogh, R. & Walker, D., eds), pp. 18–40. Kogan Page, London.

Boyd, E. and Fales, A. (1983) Reflective learning: key to learning from experience. *Journal of Humanistic Psychology*, **23**(2): 99–117.

Carper, B. (1978) Fundamental patterns of knowing in nursing. *Advances in Nursing Science*, **1**(1): 13–23.

Casement, P. (1985) *On Learning from the Patient*. Routledge, London.

Conway, J. (1996) *Nursing Expertise and Advanced Practice*. Quay Books, London.

Fay, B. (1987) *Critical Social Science*. Polity Press, Cambridge.

Freshwater, D. (2000) Cross currents: against cultural narration. *Journal of Advanced Nursing*, **32**: 481–4.

Freshwater, D. (2002) *Therapeutic Nursing: Improving Patient Care through Reflection*. Sage, London.

Freshwater, D. (2003) *Counselling Skills for Nurses, Midwives and Health Visitors*. Open University Press, Buckingham.

Freshwater, D. and Rolfe, G. (2001) Critical reflexivity: A politically and ethically engaged research method for nursing. *NT Research*, **6**(1): 526–37.

Huxley, A. (1959) *The Doors of Perception/Heaven and Hell*. Penguin Books, Harmondsworth.

Johns, C. (1995) Framing learning through reflection within Carper's ways of knowing in nursing. *Journal of Advanced Nursing*, **22**: 226–34.

Johns, C. (2002) *Guided Reflection: Advancing Practice*. Blackwell Publishing, Oxford.

Johns, C. (2004a) *Becoming a Reflective Practitioner*, 2nd edn. Blackwell Publishing, Oxford.

Johns, C. (2004b) Balancing the winds. Unpublished.

Johns, C. (2004c) *Being Mindful, Easing Suffering: Reflections on Palliative Care*. Jessica Kingsley, London.

Jones, B. and Jones, G. (1996) *Earth Dance Drum: A Celebration of Life*. Commune-a-Key, Salt Lake City.

Joyce, S. (1984) Dynamic disequilibrium: the intelligence of growth. *Theory into Practice*, **24**: 26–34.

Levine, B. (1986) *Who Dies? An Investigation of Conscious Living and Conscious Dying*. Gateway Books, Bath.

Mayeroff, M. (1971) *On Caring*. Harper Perennial, New York.

Mezirow, J. (1981) A critical theory of adult learning and education. *Adult Education,* **32**(1): 3–24.

Newman, M. (1994) *Health as Expanding Consciousness.* National League for Nursing, New York.

Prigogine, I. (1980) *From Being to Becoming.* WH Freeman, San Francisco.

Rolfe, G., Freshwater, D. and Jasper, M. (2001) *Critical Reflection for Nursing and the Helping Professions: A User's Guide.* Palgrave, Basingstoke.

Schön, D. (1983) *The Reflective Practitioner.* Avebury Press, Aldershot.

Schön, D. (1987) *Educating the Reflective Practitioner.* Jossey-Bass, San Francisco.

Sogyal (1992) *The Tibetan Book of Living and Dying.* Rider, London.

Souter, J. (2003) Using a model for structured reflection on palliative care nursing: exploring the challenges raised. *International Journal of Palliative Nursing,* **9**(1): 6–12.

White, J. (1995) Patterns of knowing: review, critique, and update. *Advances in Nursing Science,* **17**(4): 73–86.

Wilber, K. (1996) *Up from Eden: A Transpersonal View of Human Evolution,* 2nd edn. Quest Books, Wheaton, IL.

Woods, M. (2003) Using reflection in the care of a patient with lymphoedema. *British Journal of Nursing,* **12**(14): 865–70.

Young, A. (1976) *The Reflexive Universe: Evolution of Consciousness.* Robert Briggs, San Francisco.

Chapter 2

Evidence, Memory and Truth: Towards a Deconstructive Validation of Reflective Practice

Gary Rolfe

Validity and incommensurability

Research, in its broadest sense, is 'a study or experiment aimed at the discovery, interpretation, or application of facts, theories, or laws' (*New Penguin English Dictionary* 2000). If we regard reflection as a way of generating data about the world of nursing practice, then it might with some justification be regarded as a research method akin to the interview, the questionnaire and participant observation. However, most advocates of reflection view it as more than simply a data collection method; indeed, some would argue that it is a research paradigm in its own right, complete with its own perspective on the role of the reflective researcher, the relationship of reflective research to practice, and the criteria by which reflective research studies are to be judged. If we accept this view of reflection as a paradigm for collecting, judging, making sense of and applying knowledge, then reflective practice stands in the same relationship to reflection as does evidence-based practice to the randomised controlled trial (RCT). Just as the RCT is generally regarded as the gold standard for generating and evaluating knowledge for evidence-based practice, so reflection is the gold standard for generating and evaluating knowledge for reflective practice. Seen in this way, then, evidence-based practice and reflective practice are parallel philosophies about how nursing should be practised, each with self-contained but very different criteria for conducting, evaluating and applying research findings.

As Wittgenstein (1953), Kuhn (1962) and Lyotard (1988) have all pointed out, different paradigms, discourses or language games[1] are largely incommensurate. In other words, we cannot apply the rules and criteria from one to another in any meaningful way; it makes no sense to judge the findings of a reflective diary by its sample size, any more than it does to judge the findings

---

[1] For the purposes of this chapter, these three terms will be used in a narrow and more or less interchangeable sense to mean a particular view about the composition, construction, validation and dissemination of knowledge.

of an RCT by whether data saturation has been achieved. The paradigms are simply not interchangeable. Each is internally coherent but externally incompatible with the other.

This incommensurability between different research paradigms has generally been recognised and respected in the social sciences. For example, Walker (1985, pp. 15–16), writing about the qualitative and quantitative research paradigms, observed that:

> The two traditions reflect fundamentally different epistemologies concerning the sort of knowledge about the social world it is possible to achieve and different philosophies as to the nature of man.

However, whereas most social researchers would regard themselves as subscribing to either one paradigm or the other, many nurse researchers have tried to straddle both camps. Thus, for Chapman (1991, p. 39):

> Quantitative and qualitative methodologies are in fact just two different approaches to data collection and analysis and not two different philosophies of life.

Despite the desire of many nurse researchers to mix and match paradigms, most philosophers of science recognise that they *are* precisely two different philosophies of life, each with its own criteria for judging the validity of the research study. Any attempt to combine two paradigms can therefore only happen if the values and criteria of one are subordinated to the other.

Lyotard (1988, p. xi) refers to this as a *differend*, which he defines as 'a case of conflict, between (at least two) parties, that cannot be equitably resolved for lack of a rule applicable to both arguments'. For example, a dispute between a qualitative researcher and a quantitative researcher over what counts as a valid study can be settled either by applying the validity criteria of quantitative research (such as a large and randomly selected sample) or by applying the criteria of qualitative research (such as a purposively selected sample). Since each set of criteria is correct within its own paradigm but will be found lacking within the other paradigm, the argument can never be won through debate, but only by the application of power. In other words, the validity criteria that are eventually adopted will be those of the dominant paradigm, which in nursing is the positivist approach of evidence-based practice and the RCT.

This imposition of positivist values across the whole of nursing research can be seen in statements by eminent nurse researchers such as:

> There is of course a place for qualitative methods, but such research needs to use a rigorous approach *and should be linked to quantitative methodologies . . . for it to have any meaning.*
>
> (Gournay & Ritter, 1997, p. 442, my italics)

In further elucidating what they mean by 'a rigorous approach', Gournay & Ritter later added:

> We do not accept that scientific rigour is achieved by an interviewer who has not undergone interobserver reliability testing, or by validity testing that does not . . .

include test–retest data, or by use of terms such as 'symbolic interactionalism' in an article that makes no reference to Mead.

(Gournay & Ritter, 1998, p. 228)

Interobserver reliability and test–retest reliability are both criteria of quantitative research instruments, and have little or no meaning for qualitative researchers. Indeed, it is difficult even to imagine how we might go about measuring the interobserver reliability of an in-depth interview or the test–retest reliability of a set of observational field notes. Furthermore, it seems rather one-sided to expect all studies employing symbolic interactionalism to reference G.H. Mead when no one expects studies using RCTs to reference Ronald Fisher as one of the founders of the randomised controlled trial. To repeat my earlier point, the only way of combining two incommensurable paradigms is for one to be subsumed into the other, and in nursing this usually means that qualitative methodologies have to conform to the validity criteria of the dominant evidence-based positivist paradigm.

We can also see the same phenomenon occurring with reflection and reflective practice. We might expect that, as a paradigm in its own right, reflection would demonstrate its validity by adherence to its own criteria such as verisimilitude and intersubjectivity. However, there have recently been a number of calls for reflection to fall into line and justify itself according to the criteria of the dominant paradigm of evidence-based practice. Thus, Mackintosh (1998, p. 556) criticised reflective practice for not conforming to the values of the evidence-based practice paradigm:

> Much of the published evidence regarding [reflection's] impact on clinical practice appears to be based on personal anecdote and again, evidence in support of its impact on patient care is of a mainly qualitative and descriptive nature.

Even *supporters* of reflective practice have been seduced into critiquing it from the perspective of evidence-based practice and the RCT. Thus, Atkins & Murphy (1994, p. 50), while acknowledging that reflection 'does seem to have real potential for nursing practice', cautioned that 'there is as yet little research to support the use of reflection'. This observation completely misses the point that reflection *is itself* a form of research. Furthermore, it leaves reflective practitioners in the rather ludicrous position of having to carry out RCTs in order to justify their belief that knowledge obtained from reflection is of more relevance to nursing practice than knowledge from RCTs.

What, then, is to be done? If all judgements about validity are made according to the criteria of the dominant paradigm of evidence-based practice and its gold-standard methodology of the RCT, then reflection will find itself forever languishing at the bottom of the hierarchy of evidence on which practice is to be based, and reflective practitioners will be forced to justify themselves according to criteria which they regard as inappropriate. As Lyotard (1988, p. xi) pointed out:

> A wrong results from the fact that the rules of the genre of discourse by which one judges are not those of the judged genre or genres of discourse.

A wrong has resulted which is very difficult to correct. The problem is that any justification of reflective practice on its own validity criteria is likely to be dismissed as poor scholarship. How is the reflective practitioner to advocate for subjectivity and contextuality when such validity measures are viewed by the dominant discourse as evidence of poor research design? Furthermore, any defence of reflective practice from within the dominant discourse itself is likely to fail simply because the validity criteria of positivism do not apply to reflection. Once the reflective practitioner starts to make her work more objective and less contextualised, it is no longer valid by its own criteria; indeed, it is no longer true reflective practice.

But if reflection cannot challenge the dominant discourse from either inside or outside that discourse, what can be done? Lyotard's solution lies in *paralogy*, 'in which the point is not to reach agreement but *to undermine from within* the very framework in which the previous "normal science" has been conducted' (Lyotard 1984, p. xix, my italics). In other words, before reflection can be fully accepted as valid on its own terms, the validity claims of the dominant discourse must be subverted from within; that is, evidence-based practice must be undermined *by its own rules and criteria*. This subversion from within, this turning back of the rules of a discourse in order to undermine that very discourse, is precisely what Jacques Derrida had in mind when he postulated the strategy of deconstruction.

Deconstruction is . . .

Before we can employ deconstruction in order to demonstrate the validity of reflection, we must first attempt to understand what Derrida meant by it. This task is not as simple as it might first appear. One of the difficulties that many readers have with deconstruction is its slipperiness, its unwillingness to be pinned down and precisely defined. We can see its elusive nature in Derrida's constant refusal to offer a definition:

> . . . deconstruction doesn't consist in a set of theorems, axioms, tools, rules, techniques, methods . . . There is no deconstruction, deconstruction has no specific object.

> (Derrida 1996, p. 218)

> Deconstruction is not a method and cannot be transformed into one.

> (Derrida 1991, p. 273)

> It must also be made clear that deconstruction is not even an act or an operation.

> (Derrida 1991, p. 273)

> What is deconstruction? Nothing, of course!

> (Derrida 1991, p. 275)

We might be forgiven for thinking that Derrida is simply being elusive; that in refusing to define deconstruction he is merely playing a rather too clever intellectual game. However, we can perhaps get an insight into what he is attempting to convey through the above quotations if we look at one of the very few instances where he *does* provide some sort of clue about deconstruction:

> . . . perhaps deconstruction would consist, if at least it did consist, in . . . deconstructing, dislocating, displacing, disarticulating, disjointing, putting 'out of joint' the authority of the 'is'.

> (Derrida 1995, p. 25)

Here we have both the key to deconstruction and also the key to Derrida's reluctance to define it any further. Deconstruction aims to put out of joint, to 'disarticulate', the authority of the 'is'. That is to say, it refuses to take at face value any statement of the type '*x* is *y*', for example caring *is* the essence of nursing, or the randomised controlled trial *is* the gold standard of evidence. We might note in passing that in his early writing, Derrida (1976) gets around the problem of the authority of the 'is' by putting the word 'under erasure' (*sous rature*), that is, by writing is̶. By simultaneously writing the word 'is' and crossing it out, Derrida is conceding the need to employ it in order to communicate, but without necessarily accepting its usual meaning or inference.

Perhaps we can now understand Derrida's reluctance to define deconstruction, since deconstruction is not immune from its own stance of incredulity. To make any statement of the kind 'Deconstruction is . . .' would be to reject its own basic tenet of challenging the authority of the 'is'. Deconstruction must, of necessity then, remain loose and elusive. Similarly, we have seen that Derrida is reluctant to offer any rules, guidelines, tools, techniques or methods for deconstruction. Deconstruction i̶s̶ nothing; and yet it is clearly more than nothing. There is something in deconstruction; it suggests a way of getting under the skin of a discourse, of rooting out its inconsistencies and aporias. However, it is a 'something' that cannot be described, a something that can only be demonstrated. This chapter therefore offers a number of demonstrations of deconstruction in nursing. It takes as its focus three critiques of reflective practice from the dominant discourse of evidence-based practice. In particular, it attempts to demonstrate how the critiques of reflective practice can be turned back on the discourse from which they emanated; how in critiquing reflective practice, the dominant scientific discourse of nursing is also critiquing itself. As Lyotard (1988) suggested, it is only through paralogy, by undermining the dominant discourse of evidence-based practice from within, that politically weaker discourses such as reflection can be heard on their own terms. In order to demonstrate the validity of reflection, we must first show how the very criticisms directed by the dominant discourse towards reflective practice apply equally to evidence-based practice itself.

Evidence

I will begin with what is probably the most common critique of reflective practice. A number of writers have questioned the evidence base of reflection, with Carroll *et al.* (2002, p. 38) summarising this concern: 'Within the literature, there appears to be a dearth of empirical evidence supporting the usefulness of reflective practice in clinical care.' They add as a caveat that 'there is a need for rigorous research that provides evidence regarding the effectiveness of reflection and reflective practice in nursing.'

There are at least two ways of responding to this criticism. First, we might ask why 'empirical evidence' is associated exclusively with 'rigorous research', and why it is so important to justify reflective practice in this way. *Empirical evidence is literally evidence 'originating in or based on observation, experience or experiment rather than theory' (New Penguin English Dictionary* 2000). Clearly, then, the evidence derived from reflection itself can be said to be empirical, as is the evidence from casual observation. However, by associating empirical evidence with 'rigorous research', Carroll *et al.* are clearly implying a far narrower definition of what counts as the evidence base for practice. Evidence, for them, comes only from research, and probably from only particular kinds of research. As we saw earlier, Mackintosh (1998, p. 556) criticises reflective practice because

> Much of the published evidence regarding the model's impact on clinical practice appears to be based on personal anecdote, and again, evidence in support of its impact on patient care is of a mainly qualitative and descriptive nature.

In order for reflection to be an acceptable basis for practice, 'hard' evidence from quantitative research is required. As Mackintosh (1998) is quick to point out, this 'hard' empirical evidence is lacking. The problem, however, is that neither is there any hard evidence to support evidence-based practice. This rather embarrassing failure of evidence-based practice (EBP) to meet its own criteria was first noted by the Evidence-Based Medicine Working Group (1992), and later by Trinder and Reynolds (2000, p. 213), supporters of EBP, who admit:

> . . . it has not escaped the notice of either critics or champions [of EBP] that there is not, nor is likely to be, any empirical evaluation of the effectiveness of evidence-based practice itself. The lack of any empirical justification for the approach has meant that advocates have relied upon intuitive claims . . .

The superior validity of so-called evidence-based practice (that is, practice based on the evidence of research) over reflective practice is thus an act of faith of the very kind that evidence-based practice claims to reject. Indeed, it is no more or less valid than the intuitive claims advocated by reflective practitioners. It is perhaps a little ironic, then, that whilst hard empirical approaches such as EBP are condemning reflection for being based on introspection and intuition, it turns out that the only evidence for EBP is that very same introspection and intuition. The so-called experts of evidence-based practice tell us that we should reject the authority of the so-called experts in favour of the findings of research. And so we do, not thinking to question the experts who are telling us not to trust experts. Mackintosh is right to point out that the evidence in support of reflective practice is mainly of a qualitative and descriptive nature, but the same is clearly true of the evidence in support of evidence-based practice.

The second way of responding to the criticism that reflective practice is not research-based is to look with a critical eye at the very meaning of the word 'evidence'. 'Evidence: an outward sign, an indication; something, especially a fact, that gives proof or reasons for believing or agreeing with something, e.g. by a court to arrive at the truth' (*New Penguin English Dictionary* 2000). The word is derived from the Latin *ex videns*, meaning 'from what is seen'. Evidence, then, is the outwardly visible sign of an event, an indication that an event has taken place. This original meaning, in which 'evidence' is evidence *from* or evidence *of*, has more recently been supplemented by a second meaning; evidence *for*. This newer usage of the term is, strictly speaking, incorrect. When we talk of evidence *for* war or evidence *for* practice, we are not implying some kind of empirical link between the evidence and the action, but rather an ideological link. To say that there is evidence *of* the existence of weapons of mass destruction is to make a statement of empirical fact; the weapons have been seen, tested and photographed. To say that those weapons are evidence *for* war is to make a statement of belief or ideology; the weapons might or might not constitute a reason for war, depending on your views and beliefs.

Similarly, to say that there is evidence *from* a well conducted randomised controlled trial (RCT) is to make a statement of empirical fact; it is to accept the accuracy of the findings of the study and their generalisation to a wider population. However, to say that these findings constitute evidence *for* practice is to make a statement of belief or ideology that the findings from RCTs constitute a gold standard of data collection on which to base practice. Evidence-based practice takes advantage of the confusion surrounding these two quite distinct meanings of the word, which continues to convey an air of scientific, objective, empirical authority, even when being employed in its second(ary) ideological sense. When the Prime Minister speaks of 'evidence for war with Iraq', he is attempting to invoke an objective imperative, as though the link between weapons of mass destruction and military action is logical rather than ideological. Similarly, when researchers refer to the findings of RCTs as evidence for practice, they are also invoking an objective imperative, as though the link between research findings and practice based on those findings is logical rather than ideological.

However, if we accept that evidence *of* is empirically and logically stronger than evidence *for*, then ironically, evidence *of* practice in the form of naturalistic research and reflection-on-action has closer links with practice than evidence *for* practice in the form of non-naturalistic, decontextualised, experimental research.

Memory

A second critique of reflection, voiced by Newell (1992) and Reece Jones (1995), is its susceptibility to 'fallibility of recall' (Newell 1992); in other words, these critics are concerned that when I reflect, my memory might be playing tricks on me. As Reece Jones (1995, p. 787) adds, 'This raises questions about one's use of reflection: whether it reflects the incident as it actually happened or the biased version of the event.' Now clearly, memory is an essential component of reflection, which by definition entails recalling experiences after they have happened. And there is, of course, little doubt that my memory deceives me. All the time. It deceives me when I am reflecting; it deceives me when I am researching, it deceives me when I am being researched, it deceives me when I am writing. Let us take as an example the research interview, which is one of the most clear-cut cases of the distortions introduced by memory. The interviewee is being asked to recall events from the past; her thoughts, feelings, attitudes are either dredged up from her memory into consciousness during the interview, or else she formulates attitudes there and then, but based on prior experiences. This alone should alert us to the fact that research can be just as susceptible to fallibilities of memory as reflection; however, there are at least two other memories at play here.

First, there is the memory of the researcher. The researcher is interacting with the interviewee, pushing the interview in particular directions, responding on the spot to replies to earlier questions, making choices about which leads to follow up and which to return to later, *if she remembers.* And it is also memory that partly determines which lines of inquiry to follow and which to drop, since, for Freud and the psychoanalysts, it is our suppressed and repressed memories that unconsciously determine many of our conscious choices. An interviewee tells me that her dog has died. 'We'll come back to that later,' I tell her, unaware of the unconscious resistance being stirred up in my own mind due to the repressed memories of the death of my own dog when I was 5 years old. We never do come back to it; somehow, the time is taken up with other issues.

Second, there is the 'memory' of the technical devices being used to record the interview. The tape, the computer memory chips, the pen and paper. Tape recorders and computers do not suffer from quite the same problems; if microprocessors have an unconscious mind, they do not appear to let it interfere with the storage and retrieval of data. The problems here are concerned largely with the storage medium itself: tape introduces interference which can distort the message, typists mishear and mistranscribe the message into computer memory. And perhaps ironically, it is the lack of the ability to interpret (either consciously or unconsciously) that compounds the problem. The human mind compensates for loss of information: if the sound level is low or muffled, the human brain can fill in the gaps, can create meaning out of silence. The computer memory, on the other hand, remembers only the silence, the gap, the missing word that the typist could not quite make out. And when I do finally come to analyse this incomplete data, I have to rely on my own memory to fill in the gaps, to recall what was actually said during the interview, or at least what my memory would like me to believe was actually said.

But we should not think that quantitative research is any less susceptible to distortion caused by memory. Items on closed questionnaires and attitude scales might well be coded in a seemingly objective numerical format and stored on a computer, but they still require the respondent to delve into her organic and all too fallible memory to retrieve the responses in the first place. When I ask a research subject to respond to a Likert scale statement such as 'Education is a good thing', her coded response of '2' refers to the verbal statement 'partially agree', which in turn refers to a judgement based on an almost infinite amount of data stored in her brain, some of which is fully accessible, some partly accessible, but most totally unavailable to her. The seemingly objective numerical score conceals a subjective judgement based on an unreliable memory.

It would appear, then, that all of the evidence on which we base our practice is contaminated by memory, whether that evidence derives from reflection or from empirical research. But further, the very act of applying evidence to practice entails yet more of Newell's 'fallibility of recall'. Our reflections might be written up in a diary, the research findings might be published in a journal paper, but at the moment that we are confronted with a clinical decision, all we have is what we remember of this evidence; all we have is our fallible memory. Our clinical decision is based not on ten impeccably con-ducted randomised controlled trials, but on our recollections of the main findings of those RCTs. Unless we retreat back to the library every time we make a clinical decision, we are totally dependent on our memory. So Newell is right to identify fallibility of recall as a factor in collecting and applying the evidence from reflective practice, but it is equally a factor in collecting and applying all forms of evidence.

Truth

In a paper entitled 'Telling lies: faking the story', Cox (2002) tells the story of Alice. Alice is a busy nurse who, when asked to write a reflective assignment for a course she was taking, constructed a 'story' of a patient with bipolar affective disorder based partly on her own life experiences and partly on her existing theoretical knowledge:

> Alice reflected. She looked into the mirror and thought, 'This is pretty good. No one will know that I have faked the story.'

> (Cox 2002, p. 113)

Cox is concerned that students are faking it, that they are writing 'a mixture of truth and fiction', and that the lesson they are learning is: 'Distort the truth. Distort the experience. Give the teacher or clinical supervisor something that is interesting to read . . . Not reality, but a construction of the imagination'

(Cox 2002). How are we to know, then, if we are being deceived by a lie, by a 'fake' reflective account, and what is the student learning from constructing such an account apart from how to cheat the system?

There are a number of points to be made about this critique of reflection. The first and perhaps the most obvious is that Cox has employed a story which is, by her own admission, 'a mixture of truth and fiction' in order to criticise the student for writing a story. The worry for Cox is that students are learning to distort the truth, to distort the experience in order to give the reader something interesting, but isn't that exactly what Cox is doing in her own story? Or perhaps Cox is relating a real event, a 'truth' rather than a 'lie'. But a closer inspection of the story reveals that this is unlikely to be the case. The story is written from a 'third person omniscient' point of view: from the eye of God. The narrator is able to see inside Alice's head, to read her thoughts, the narrator (Cox) is able to tell us things about Alice that only Alice herself could know. So perhaps the story is autobiographical; perhaps Alice is actually Cox; perhaps Cox is relating a story from her own experience as a student. Perhaps. But that does not make the story any less of a lie; Cox would still be distorting the story in order to make a point, in order to make it more interesting to the reader. Whichever way we look at it, this story is a fiction, a fake. Cox is using fiction in order to make a case against fiction.

But let us look more closely at what Cox is claiming: that students are writing 'a mixture of truth and fiction'; that they are distorting the truth; and ultimately, that they are 'telling lies and faking the story'. Clearly, she is drawing on a number of dichotomies here: between the true and the false, between truth and lies, between fact and fiction, between the real and the fake:

truth   lies
real   fake
fact   fiction
true   false

Unfortunately, she is becoming confused over these pairs of polar opposites, she is muddling them up, assuming that they are more or less interchangeable. Alice is telling lies, which means that she is not telling the truth. Her story is fake rather than real, fiction rather than fact, therefore it is false rather than true; facts are true, therefore fiction must be false. Alice's story is thus 'a mixture of truth and fiction', as though these two terms also form a dichotomy, a pair of polar opposites.

However, it is not at all self-evident that fiction is the opposite of truth; that fiction is necessarily false. The linguist Noam Chomsky (1988, p. 159) tells us that:

> It is quite possible – overwhelmingly probable, one might guess – that we will always learn more about human life and human personality from novels than from scientific psychology.

Fiction can be a valuable source of knowledge, of truth. As Foucault (1980, p. 193) adds:

I am well aware that I have never written anything but fictions. I do not mean to say, however, that truth is therefore absent. It seems to me that the possibility exists for fiction to function in truth, for a fictional discourse to induce the effects of truth.

Clearly, the dichotomy of truth on the one hand and fiction on the other is suspect. Worse still, it is based on a linguistic error. When Cox suggests that fiction is a distortion of the truth, that fiction is untrue, she is confusing the word 'fictional' with the word 'fictitious'. 'Fictional' means simply 'from fiction', which in turn is derived from the Latin *fingere*, meaning 'to shape or construct'. There is no implication here of lies or deceit, simply of creating something. On the other hand, 'fictitious' means false or feigned, and is probably what Cox really means when she accuses students of writing fictional accounts. But, of course, Cox's failure to distinguish between the two words destroys her entire argument. Whilst she might be excused for criticising Alice for writing a fictitious (that is, a deceitful) account, there is nothing *inherently* false or untrue about it. A fictitious (deceitful) story, which is also a fictional (made up) story, can still convey truths and can still be learnt from, as Chomsky and Foucault suggest above. Just because Alice has lied to her tutor about the origins of her story does not necessarily mean that the story is itself a lie; that it does not speak the truth. Alice's story was completely fictitious and partially fictional, and yet it also 'induced the effects of truth' as Foucault put it, and it is possible, as Chomsky said, that Alice learnt more from writing her fictitious/fictional story than she would have done from writing a traditional 'true' textbook assignment on bipolar affective disorder. Similarly, Cox's story about Alice was also fictitious and was perhaps at least partly fictional, and yet it also 'induced the effects of truth' and perhaps allowed us to learn more about reflection than a traditional textbook account would have done.

Conclusion

This chapter has attempted to defend and promote the validity of reflection by providing some examples of how the dominant discourse of scientific evidence-based practice is open to many of the very critiques that it directs at less powerful discourses such as reflective practice. It has argued that most discourses are internally consistent and can only be challenged by stepping outside their own rules and conventions in what Lyotard referred to as paralogy. The gold-standard status of the RCT cannot be challenged from within the discourse of EBP, since that discourse *defines* the RCT as providing the best possible evidence for practice. The only way that the self-defined gold-standard status of the RCT can be critiqued is by challenging it from *outside* the dominant discourse. The problem, however, is that such challenges are easily dismissed. By defining reflection as a weak form of evidence, or even as not evidence at all, the arguments of reflective practitioners are diminished in status. Thus, reflective practice is easily rejected as not being based on the findings of RCTs, even though, as Trinder & Reynolds (2000) observed, the status of the RCT as providing the best evidence for practice is not itself empirically founded but is accepted as *self-evidently* true.

The problem for discourses such as reflective practice is that the dominant discourse of EBP has the power to determine what will and will not be taken as self-evident in the discipline of nursing, and that once something is accepted as self-evident, it is very difficult to challenge. Deconstruction gets around this problem by turning the critiques aimed by EBP at other discourses back on to EBP itself. It does not attempt to apply the tenets and criteria of reflection to EBP, but rather demonstrates that EBP falls short of its *own* tenets and criteria. It points out that the justification of being 'self-evident' is itself rejected by EBP as a form of evidence, and that, in effect, evidence-based practice is no more based on evidence than the forms of practice it seeks to replace.

The self-proclaimed validity of EBP can only be achieved by diminishing the validity claims of other incompatible discourses such as reflection. Consequently, the validity of reflection as a source of knowledge for nursing practice can only be promoted by deconstructing the dominant discourse of evidence-based practice in order to show that *no* discourse is able to make the kind of sweeping validity claims that EBP has attempted in the past.

Postscript: deconstruction ~~is~~ . . .

I claimed at the start of this chapter that deconstruction cannot be defined or even adequately explained; it can only be demonstrated. I then offered three examples of deconstruction in action in order to question the status of EBP as self-evidently valid. What, then, can we learn about deconstruction from these examples? We can see, first, that it is best employed to challenge critiques made by the dominant discourse against less powerful discourses. And it does so *not* by denying the charges laid against the less powerful discourse, but by turning them back against the dominant discourse from which they originated. So, for example, deconstruction accepts that reflective practice is not supported by 'hard' research evidence; that it is open to the distortions of memory; and that it can sometimes consist in little more than fictional and/or fictitious stories. But then it points out that evidence-based practice is also not supported by hard research evidence; that the generation and application of research findings to practice is itself open to the distortions of memory; and that critics of reflective practice are just as capable of telling stories in order to make their case.

Second, deconstruction is concerned with language and the way that it is often distorted by the dominant discourse to its own ends. So, for example, it demonstrates how the word 'evidence' has been used to provide a logical, empirical facade to research-based practice, and how the original etymological meaning of evidence links it more closely to reflection than to experimental research.

Third, deconstruction attempts to break down dichotomies in which one term is favoured over its opposite by the dominant discourse. The most obvious example is the way in which evidence-based practice has been set up in opposition to reflective practice:

Evidence-based practice	*Reflective practice*
based on hard research	based on personal anecdote and intuition
objective and unbiased	biased due to fallible human memory
based on truth	based on fiction

The aim of deconstruction is not to *reverse* the dichotomy, not to claim that reflection, intuition, memory and fiction are better than their counterparts, but to show that the dichotomy is itself flawed; that there *is* no dichotomy. So, for example, deconstruction demonstrates that fiction is *not* the opposite of truth; that a story can be both fictional and true; that it can even be both *fictitious* and true. Ultimately, then, the dichotomy between evidence-based practice and reflective practice is also flawed. Intuition and reflection are not opposed to evidence, nor are they inferior forms of evidence. 'Hard' research and 'soft' intuition have more in common than perhaps either the evidence-based practitioner or the reflective practitioner would care to admit.

Deconstruction is therefore perhaps not such a negative term as its name suggests (as one critic unkindly put it, deconstruction puts the con in destruction). If deconstruction is concerned with destruction at all, it is with the destruction of the walls that have been built between the self-proclaimed dominant discourses and the other discourses that they seek to suppress. Deconstruction does not proclaim that all discourses are equal, but, on the contrary, that all are different and must be judged according to their own criteria. And ultimately, it seeks to demonstrate that any attempt to make judgements according to the standards of the dominant discourse (evidence, memory, truth) can simply be turned back on the dominant discourse itself.

References

Atkins, S. and Murphy, K. (1994) Reflective practice. *Nursing Standard*, 8(39): 49–56.

Carroll, M., Curtis, L., Higgins, A., Nicholl, H., Redmond, R. and Timmins, F. (2002) Is there a place for reflective practice in the nursing curriculum? *Nurse Education in Practice*, **2**: 13–20.

Chapman, J. (1991) Research – what it is and what it is not. In *Nursing: A Knowledge Base for Practice* (Perry, A. & Jolley, M. eds), pp. 28–51. Edward Arnold, London.

Chomsky, N. (1988) *Language and the Problems of Knowledge*. MIT Press, Cambridge, MA.

Cox, C. (2002) Telling lies: faking the story. In *Enhancing the Practice Experience* (Cox, C. ed.), pp. 108–16. Nursing Praxis International, Bournemouth.

Derrida, J. (1976) *Of Grammatology*. Johns Hopkins University Press, Baltimore, MD.

Derrida, J. (1991) Letter to a Japanese friend. In *A Derrida Reader: Reading Between the Blinds* (Kamuf, P., ed.), pp. 270–6. Harvester Wheatsheaf, New York.

Derrida, J. (1995) The time is out of joint. In *Deconstruction is/in America* (Haverkamp, A., ed.), pp. 14–41. New York University Press, New York.

Derrida, J. (1996) *As if* I were dead: an interview with Jacques Derrida. In *Applying: To Derrida* (Brannigan, J., Robbins, R. & Wolfreys, J. eds), pp. 212–27. Macmillan, London.

Evidence-Based Medicine Working Group (1992) Evidence-based medicine: a new approach to teaching the practice of medicine. *Journal of the American Medical Association*, **268**(17): 2420–5.

Foucault, M. (1980) *Power/Knowledge, Selected Interviews and Other Writings 1972–1977*. Harvester Press, Brighton.

Gournay, K. and Ritter, S. (1997) What future for research in mental health nursing? *Journal of Psychiatric and Mental Health Nursing*, **4**: 441–6.

Gournay, K. and Ritter, S. (1998) What future for research in mental health nursing: rejoinder to Parsons, Beech and Rolfe. *Journal of Psychiatric and Mental Health Nursing*, **5**: 227–35.

Kuhn, T. (1962) *The Structure of Scientific Revolutions*. University of Chicago Press, Chicago IL.

Lyotard, J-F. (1984) *The Postmodern Condition: A Report on Knowledge*. Manchester University Press, Manchester.

Lyotard, J-F. (1988) *The Differend: Phrases in Dispute*. University of Minnesota Press, Minneapolis, MN.

Mackintosh, C. (1998) Reflection: a flawed strategy for the nursing profession? *Nurse Education Today*, **18**: 553–7.

New Penguin English Dictionary (2000) Ed. R. Allen. Penguin Books Ltd, London.

Newell, R. (1992) Anxiety, accuracy and reflection: the limits of professional development. *Journal of Advanced Nursing*, **17**(6): 364–70.

Reece Jones, P. (1995) Hindsight bias in reflective practice: an empirical investigation. *Journal of Advanced Nursing*, **21**: 783–8.

Trinder, L. and Reynolds, S. (2000) *Evidence-Based Practice: A Critical Appraisal*. Blackwell Science, Oxford.

Walker, R. (1985) *Applied Qualitative Research*. Gower Publishing, Aldershot.

Wittgenstein, L. (1953) *Philosophical Investigations*. Basil Blackwell, Oxford.

Chapter 3

Living Relational Ethics in Health Care

Bernie Pauly and Susan James

Relational ethics begins with the assumption that ethical practice occurs within relationships and that relationships are a source of moral knowing (Bergum 1998; Austin *et al.* 2003; Bergum 2004).

> A relational ethic stimulates a fundamental shift in our thinking about ethics. There is a move from concentration on solving the ethical 'problem' to asking the ethical question. The focus shifts from attention to the person as an individual (that is, a solitary bearer of rights) to recognition of the person as an interdependent agent (autonomous but situated in community with others, and thereby connected to others).
>
> (Austin *et al.*, p. 45)

Relational ethics brings a new perspective to health care ethics that builds upon and extends to other forms of ethical theory such as principle-, virtue- and rights-based theories. In a relational ethic, the practitioner builds on traditional knowledge of ethical theories and principles while moving to a greater understanding of the meaning of the situation through relationship with another.

The Relational Ethics Project (1993–2001), with funding from the Social Sciences and Humanities Research Council of Canada led by Vangie Bergum and John Dossetor, was undertaken with the purpose of illuminating the meaning of ethical commitments within health care relationships in everyday situations (Austin *et al.* 2003). Health care scenarios were explored in order to develop a clearer understanding of ethical commitments within relationships and of relational ethics that would build upon traditional knowledge of ethical theories and principles. In the initial phase of the project, core themes emerged which were viewed as central to a theory of relational ethics. The themes included mutual respect, engagement, embodied knowledge and attention to the environment. In the second phase, the goal was to explore these themes in particular practice contexts (mental health, genetic counselling and health care provider relationships). Both authors were members of the interdisciplinary Relational Ethics Research Group.

At the beginning of the Relational Ethics Project, it was recognised that we needed to bring living examples to our work together as an interdisciplinary research team. A variety of approaches (videos, photographs, personal stories, literature and art) were explored to help us to describe relational ethics.

Narratives, images, and drama have great potential to teach about ourselves and the nature of healthcare work, to sharpen visual sense, generate new insights and under- standings and to promote ethical awareness. In a relational ethic both the heart and the mind must be stimulated as neither mind nor emotion alone is sufficient.

(Bergum 1998, p. 2)

In this chapter a narrative between a woman and her nurse-midwife (the authors) will bring to life the meaning of relational ethics. The voices of both will explore, debate and discuss the nature of mutual respect in health care as a means for valuing and supporting cultural diversity.

The woman's story

"Three years ago I entered into a practitioner/client relationship with a nursing colleague. I was pregnant and had decided that I would like to have a midwife attend my birth. There are a number of qualified midwives within a 90-mile radius, so I did my homework and sought the opinion of other colleagues. Initially, I didn't consider Susan for the very reason that she and I were col- leagues and associates on this project. I thought it might create role confusion. However, as I completed my research the evidence was clear that she and her partner midwives were the best in the business. So I put aside my reservations and, to my surprise, she didn't hesitate when I asked her to be my midwife. It never occurred to me that she might discuss my situation with our fellow colleagues. I just knew she would not. I remember feeling a bit nervous and worried that it might seem strange or uncomfortable or that she might see me in a vulnerable or unflattering way. However, before the end of the first visit my worries evaporated. I did at times wonder in the back of mind what she might think of me as a colleague once this was over. However, I trusted her to handle the situation with the same degree of professionalism that she had displayed thus far.

As my due date approached, my husband and I made the decision that not only did we want a midwife but also we wanted a home birth. We carefully considered the statistics, the risks and the benefits. Having a home birth won hands down and Susan supported our process of decision making. I never for one moment doubted her competency. I believed she would manage the birth and any outcomes as competently as she handled every question I asked and every check-up she did. In fact, I trusted her more than my physician whose main goal seemed to be to dissuade me from having a home birth by telling me about one woman who had a dangerously low haemoglobin (less than 2) when her midwife brought her to the hospital.

When the day of the birth arrived, I called Susan and she was there. She never left my side. The most amazing part was her ability to facilitate the pro- cess of birth while allowing me to be my own guide. I would say 'I don't know what to do,' and she would make suggestions. The birth was amazing. Susan helped us to make memories through her observations and comments.

Then I began to haemorrhage. Susan gave me a herb to contract the uterus, started an IV and administered medications. When I didn't stop bleeding, she calmly told me it was time to call the doctor or go the hospital. We called the ambulance. I knew I had a retained placenta and needed a D&C. No one at the hospital seemed to understand this and I couldn't seem to tell them. The words seemed to be locked in my mind. Although I was shouting the words inside my head, I couldn't seem to express them. I'm not sure what Susan told them but the obstetrician didn't seem to appreciate my need and decided to observe me for four hours, during which time I bled and bled and bled until I needed five units of blood transfused. What went wrong: the lack of continuity, the lack of respect, or disregard for the information Susan provided? The relationship that failed was the one between providers, the system and myself, not myself and my midwife. How could the other providers not know what I knew and Susan knew?

I don't know what Susan told them, but whatever it was no one listened or took the necessary action. Susan stayed with me, soothing me, comforting me, reassuring me when I became upset. Finally, I convinced a nurse that I needed to be reassessed. I was in bad shape. They were pumping in IV fluid faster and faster each time my blood pressure fell and I lost consciousness. I must have had water in my veins. I clearly remember the ride to the OR. I knew I was in bad shape just by the number of intravenous lines and the speed at which people were moving. No waiting in the operating room: straight into the theatre. I begged for someone to talk to me. The anaesthesist said that the nurse would talk to me and she did. I will never forget waking up post-surgery with my body painfully swollen and MAST pants on to shunt the blood to the core of my body. From working in the emergency room, I knew that MAST pants are only used when someone has lost an excessive amount of blood, and providers are struggling to maintain the person's blood pressure. I will never forget that terrible night struggling to breast feed, IVs in each antecubital space. The nurse checking my IV, catheter, intake and output. 'Excuse me, I'm a person,' I felt like saying. I will never forget the nurse who touched my swollen face, disproportionate from a massive fluid shift the next day. She was the only kind one. I will never forget the lectures and reprimands: from my general practitioner, 'I knew this would happen to you'; the obstetrician, 'This didn't have to happen'; the scolding from the afternoon nurse, 'I hope you'll never do that again'.

Eight months later I saw an ER nurse who reminded me how lucky I was and how dangerous home births were. Eight months later I was still being blamed. I was the star of the urban legend of the woman who nearly died of a post-partum hemorrhage during a home birth. No one seemed to understand that it was not the home birth that nearly killed me but the wait at the hospital until someone came to their senses. The ethical violations were not in my relationship with my midwife but in my relations with other health care providers and the health care system or I should say the lack of a relationship with them. I was never real for them: I was a myth, a folk tale, an anomaly, a threat to the system. The painful part is that I was once a nurse in the emergency room. I knew the doctor and many of the nurses on call that day. I greeted them by name. They too were colleagues. I never became their client. Months later I had ER nurses tell me how well I looked considering the terrible shape I had arrived in. Where was the confidentiality? Was it easy to talk about me since they knew me as a colleague but not as a client?

It was my very relationship with Susan that led to my trust in her. The boundaries of our relationship were clearly established during my first visit with her. As the professional, she took the initiative in establishing those boundaries and as the client I appreciated this. My greatest concern in the end was how much I put her and my husband and child through. For many months I felt it was my fault. I felt I had been betrayed by my own profession, which I loved deeply. I was angry and hurting."

The nurse-midwife's story

"Bernie was not my first client who wasn't just a client. I started my midwifery practice by doing midwifery care for friends, classmates, team-mates and co-workers. One of my greatest joys was being my youngest sister's midwife for her two births. The 'new' midwives in Canada and the United States who practised outside of regulation didn't worry a lot about professional boundaries. Being a woman's midwife meant that you expected to become very close throughout the pregnancy and birthing experiences. Having a client start off as a friend or colleague just seemed to make it all easier.

When Bernie asked me about my services, I recall the excitement of realising that Bernie and Bear were expecting a baby and that this was news that had not yet been shared with most of the rest of the group. I realise that some of the concerns that are raised about intermingling professional and personal boundaries are around issues of confidentiality. Midwives say that providing care for friends and family means that they have to be a little cautious about casual conversations in family or social settings that could reveal information that is not meant to be shared. I remember waiting for a sign that Vangie or Sandy or John, our fellow team members, knew this news.

I found it interesting to enter into this relationship of being woman and midwife in the midst of a relational ethics project. We had spent hours talking about the appropriateness of emotions in professional work, the need for professional boundaries and the problems that professional boundaries create, and about needing to be open to knowing the individual and authentic in our ways of being ourselves in our professional roles. It seemed as though Bernie and I were embarking on an opportunity to walk the talk. And yet, I sometimes sensed a caution from some group members. 'What will you do if something goes wrong?' 'How comfortable will you be, making hard decisions?' 'What about the intimacy inherent in childbirth?'

And so we began our journey getting to know one another as midwife and woman. Each prenatal visit or class was an opportunity to understand what Bernie and Bear wanted for this experience and for me to reflect on my own ability to assist them to achieve that. I remember vividly the week that Bernie had a disagreement with her family doctor. I felt privileged to have shared the experience of the relational ethics work with Bernie. It helped make clear her outrage.

Bernie called to tell me she was in labour in the middle of the night. I had just hung up the phone from a call with another woman who was in early labour. It was clear that Bernie was in strong labour and needed me to come. I called the first woman back and asked her to stop labouring, that it was Bernie's turn now and that she needed to wait (and she did!). We headed off to Bernie's, full of excitement at this coming birth. All births are special, but there is a different anticipation when the woman isn't just a client. There are many memories of Bernie's labour that come to mind: the drumming music (now known as Brenna's drums), Bernie leaning over the huge cannonball posts of her bed while we put pressure on her back, eating frozen blueberries, her sister baking muffins, filling up the double sized tub, Bernie realising that Brenna was nearly born, and Bear's joy at being able to catch their daughter as Bernie pushed. I will always remember the look on Bernie's face as she sat on her bedroom floor cradling Brenna in her arms and her words 'Oh Bear, I really like her. Do you like her?' These are the moments that draw me to my work.

But, the story does not end here. Bernie's placenta was reluctant to come out. It was clear that I was going to have to intervene and ultimately advise Bernie that we should go to hospital as a fragment of placenta remained inside and Bernie was bleeding heavily and becoming shocked. The paramedics arrived and were initially hostile, but I remembered one of them from a class I had taught the year before and reminded him of our connection. Suddenly, they became friendly and cooperative. Our experience in the hospital was not pleasant. The staff were unwilling to hear my report of the events that preceded the transfer. And, although they knew Bernie as a colleague, they criticised her choice to have a home birth, implying that it was her fault that she ended up in this very grave situation. There came a point where I feared that Bernie could die. Her condition was becoming more and more critical. The physician was not in the hospital and the staff were not willing to call him. Strange thoughts go through one's mind when in such difficult situations. I recall thinking that Vangie would be pretty angry with me if one of her favourite students died while under my care. I felt helpless and invisible. Each time that I asked the nurse when they might do something to help Bernie, I received blank stares in return or was told that the doctor would be here at dinnertime. Finally, requests from all of us, midwives, family, Bernie herself, stimulated the call to the physician who ordered blood transfusions and came to do the D&C."

I often wonder about the caution, 'What will you do if something goes wrong?' If this had been another woman, would I have acted in a different way, perhaps delaying the decision to transfer, or perhaps intervening sooner? Would I have taken a different approach, perhaps just telling her that we need to go to hospital rather than providing all the information about what was happening with the bleeding and the limits of my expertise and equipment and then giving Bernie and Bear the final decision about transfer? Would I have felt more or less invisible or frustrated in the hospital? Would I still have strong memories of this whole experience?

Perhaps a midwife cannot answer these questions. By the time of birth, it can be difficult to differentiate women with whom we have had a pre-existing personal relationship from the women whom we meet for the first time early in pregnancy.

According to Bergum (2004, p. 494), 'Mutual respect arises from the reality that we are fundamentally connected to one another. Our experience of our world and of ourselves is shaped by the attitude of others towards us and by our attitude towards others.' In the Relational Ethics Research Project 'respect for one another' emerged as a central and essential theme in relational ethics. Mutual respect involves recognition, acknowledgement and appreciation of difference in power, knowledge, experience, attitudes, values and beliefs.

Susan: "One of my thoughts of what happened when we came into the emergency department was that the staff made *a priori* assumptions about you. Rather than connecting with you and Bear and me to understand this particular situation, perhaps they assumed that you were inappropriately cared for because you had a home birth. I recall the emergency physician's first 'diagnosis' that this bleeding must be coming from a severe laceration even though your 'clinical picture' was clearly pointing to other diagnoses. Perhaps they assumed that you did not want interventions because you chose a home birth. Perhaps this is the explanation for the very long wait for the intervention for which we came to the hospital. What happens when we make such strong assumptions? In some ways, you would have had better treatment if they had approached you as 'any woman' – any woman who arrived in the emergency department with heavy bleeding and signs of shock. Perhaps they believed that they were treating the individual – this individual who wants an alternative approach to her pregnancy and childbirth."

Bernie: "I've often thought that I might have been treated differently if I was a woman transferred in from a small rural hospital rather than my home. The set of assumptions about me and the amount of intervention I wanted might have been very different. It is very true that one reason that I chose a home birth was the promise of limited intervention. However, I assumed that, if I needed to be transferred, then it was for an intervention. The point is that their assumptions were right when I was at home but didn't hold true in the hospital. I recall one nurse asking me hesitantly if I would accept a blood transfusion. I remember thinking, 'Are you nuts? Of course, I'm bleeding to death here.' I wonder if anyone at the hospital was even consciously aware of the assumptions that they were making and how it was affecting their relationship with us and their decision making about my care.

Assumptions colour our relationships with others. Jean Watson (1979), in a discussion of the carative factor of altruistic humanistic values, highlights the importance of reflecting on our own values, attitudes and beliefs before engaging with a client. I would guess, the assumptions you (Susan) started with were very different from those of other providers (i.e. my physician). I think one of the assumptions I had that made a home birth acceptable was that the health care system would be there if I needed it. I never thought I would be punished because of my choice. I think that was a great shock to me. Now I know I can't count on other providers or the system if I make unpopular choices.

Relational ethics shows our connections to each other and that we are always in relation and never out of relation. We are interdependent, and the nature of respect in relational ethics is interactive and reciprocal (Bergum 2004, p. 495):

> It seems easy to speak of respect – 'I respect your wish for . . .' – yet harder to prac-
> tice the attitude of 'I respect you,' especially if I think what you do is inappropriate.

Mutual respect calls for respect for difference. As health care providers, enacting mutual respect would point to finding ways that allow us to engage and work with people even when negative judgements are provoked, on the basis that everyone is deserving of respect."

Susan: "Not only is it essential to know one's self before entering into our relations with our clients, we must also be open to hearing, seeing, respecting the values, attitudes and beliefs of others. I suspect that it is in that openness that we really learn about our selves. When another challenges what we believe or value, we could take an approach, perhaps guided by principles of autonomy, where we stop at this point, saying that it is all right for you and me to be different. Each of us has a right to self-determination and to make our own decisions. Or, we could move beyond this to try to come to some understanding of both our views. What is it about the challenge that further entrenches me in my views? What is it about my views that evokes such strong challenges? Can we find a way to work together even when we hold different values? *A priori* assumptions can act as a barrier to working together if we are so attached to our assumptions that we cannot let them go. I too assume that when we need the health care system, it will be there for us. And often it is. I assume that if I bring in my documentation on my care and give a careful report of my observations and actions, this information will be listened to and considered in the planning of the next steps in the care of the woman. Often this is what happens. But, frequently enough, the experience that I had with you in the hospital is the approach that other health care providers take when I must interface with the system. At this point in my career, I don't know why I continue to be surprised by this."

Bernie: "The attention to the attitudes, values and beliefs of ourselves and others needs to continue throughout the relationship, not just at the beginning as you identified. I think that is what Jean Watson (1988) means when she talks about the relationship being the moral end. When I enter into the relationship, I am morally obligated to understand the other even when our view differs. I think the skill of the provider is in being able to say, 'These are my views, these are my assumptions,' and try to be aware of them in the moment as they listen to the other. What are your views, your assumptions? I think we are mistaken if we seek to put our assumptions aside. I'm not sure we can ever let go of them but we can try to be aware of them in the moment and recognise them as our own. In that way we can truly listen to the other. If we cannot engage without seeing the other as the same as ourselves, we will fail to connect with the other as a person (Bergum 2004)."

Susan: "I suggest that not doing (or neglect) is also a response that occurs with the absence of relationship. In the hospital I felt powerless, invisible. Was this because there was a lack of a commitment to a relational approach to both you and me? Was this felt even more acutely in contrast to the home birth that we had just left? Or even in contrast to the paramedics who moved into a relational approach when 'invited' to remember that there was reason to recognise relations with us. Would the staff also have felt powerless in this situation? Did they feel somehow neglected or devalued because of the choice to have a care provider that they do not view as being legitimate? Or because of the choice to have a home birth? Would this perception of being devalued be even stronger when the patient/client is 'one of theirs'? How would these nurses and physicians interpret your choice? If they were basing their interpretation on generalised assumptions about the (in)competency of midwives, the (lack of) safeness in home birth, the personal characteristics of any woman who would make these choices, perhaps they assume that your choice is a slap in their faces. Does she think that care is so bad in the hospital that she would make this 'inferior' choice? Does she not like them? Does she not trust them? Perhaps they feel a need to ignore you, to punish you, to slap back."

Bernie: "I hadn't considered that they too might feel powerless. Were they thinking, 'How do we handle this situation which is very complicated because this is one of our own?' or 'The care is so wonderful here, how could she not choose to come here?' Was the difficulty the fact that my choices (midwife and home birth) were so challenging to their belief system that they were forced to neglect us in defence of the system they work within? When people make choices that challenge our belief systems to such a degree, are we forced to choose between the two?

I recall the change in attitude of the paramedic after Susan reminded him of their past relationship. He became more attentive, sensitive and understanding. He seemed to see the world from the perspective of a woman and her midwife. I asked him not to judge what had happened here. He said he wouldn't and I believed him. I remember feeling relieved, and believed that he would do everything to help us. There was a significant shift in our relation with him. Was he able for a moment to see into our world in spite of the dominant worldview? I never felt we were able to achieve this kind of relationship with the physicians and nurses at the hospital. He entered our home. We entered the hospital. He entered our turf.

We entered their turf. How can we enter each other's turf even when they are on our turf? How do we overcome feeling powerless in light of our assumptions/judgements so that we can engage rather than disengage?"

Susan: "I find your question of how we overcome feeling powerless so that we can engage rather than disengage to be one of the greatest challenges that I experience in midwifery practice. I find the level of polite or friendly engagement to be fairly easy to accomplish when entering a situation where I feel powerless. While being polite or friendly eases some of the communication challenges, this approach seldom overturns powerlessness. Sometimes, this approach actually contributes to building powerlessness. My friendliness with nurses sometimes results in a sense that I'm 'one of them' and therefore I am pulled into their own relations of powerlessness in the system. In an environment where rudeness and lack of consideration are often behaviours associated with power (and therefore knowledge and skill), politeness can be perceived as ignorance. I am reluctant to engage in those behaviours associated with power. When these behaviours come from someone not given the 'right' to express them (patient/client or care provider), we often label that person as being a problem – too noisy, too demanding, doesn't know their place, difficult. To some extent the feeling of powerlessness is internal. I have a strong sense of knowing my own strengths and limitations in my practice area: why should I feel powerless? But when I am not heard or seen, all the knowledge and skills in the world will not give me power. I wonder how women can overcome feelings of powerlessness when the structures supporting power relations are so strong."

Bernie: "I think your comments are a wonderful illustration of the difference between 'power with' and 'power over'. The perception exists that if we enter into relationships in which power is shared we will lose something. We will give up some of our power. We want to hold power because that is what the system values. Yet, for people to be autonomous and for us to support them, we have to move into a relational ethic which values power with, not power over.

According to Myra Levine (1977, p. 846):

> Ethical behavior is not the display of one's moral rectitude in times of crisis. It is the day-to-day expression of one's commitment to other persons and the ways in which human beings relate to one another in their daily interactions."

Susan: "And yet, it is times of crisis that are the biggest worry about the intermingling of boundaries and roles. I am consistently challenged: 'What will you do in a crisis?' In some ways, Myra Levine's advice, 'It is the day-to-day expression of one's commitment to other persons and the ways in which human beings relate to one another in their daily interactions,' is really the biggest issue for intermingling roles. The challenges are in being clear about not taking advantage of privileged knowledge, not making assumptions because both know one another in other circumstances, finding the day-to-day balances of these roles, finding courage and confidence, finding humility. Perhaps it is in meeting these challenges that we can find a way to be in power with rather than to be in power over.

Perhaps we could say that with relational ethics, from the perspective of mutual respect, we focus on who we are rather than what we do, that is, a way of being rather than a mode of decision making. It is not enough to assist people to make fully informed competent choices but to stay with them as they live their choices."

Bernie: "The day-to-day expression of one's commitment is critical to relational ethics and is demonstrated in our relationships. The health care practitioner is required to be self-aware and reflective of differences, not only at the beginning of the relationship but throughout the duration of the relationship. The ethical practitioner is mindful of self and others. These are some assumptions necessary for a relational ethic. What about being altruistic? The traditional notion of altruism is selflessness. However, it is possible to redefine this to be other-focused without selflessness. As Sally Gadow (1990) has pointed out in her work on existential advocacy, being other-focused is the greatest gift we give others because they can never achieve it themselves."

Susan: "And I think that being other-focused is also a gift to ourselves. If totally selfless giving or altruism is the ideal in health care, perhaps this is when we find ourselves in situations like yours where you become a legend, to be discussed in the most public and unethical ways possible. Being selfless allows us to be non-reflective, to give and give without thinking, and all the while believing that we are doing excellent work. Giving without thinking of ourselves ultimately means that we don't really think about the other to whom we give. It is only through thinking about ourselves that we come to recognise the individuality of the other. The gift that we receive is that in thinking about another, we come to learn more about ourselves. Is it selfish to see oneself reflected through another? Is it selfish to discover a deeper understanding of the multidimensional sense of who I am? Consider the memories that I have of your birth. These memories can renew my commitment to my work, to women and to myself. Each memory is a simple act, and yet each memory is a sacrament. This was your birth. These memories come to me as a gift from you."

References

Austin, W., Bergum, V. and Dossetor, J. (2003) Relational ethics: an action ethics as a foundation. In *Approaches to Ethics: Nursing beyond Boundaries* (Tschudin, V., ed.), pp. 45–52. Butterworth Heinemann, Toronto.

Bergum, V. (1998) Relational ethics: what is it? In *Touch: the Provincial Health Ethics Network*, **1**(2): 1–2.

Bergum, V. (2004) Relational ethics in nursing. In *Toward a Moral Horizon: Nursing Ethics for Leadership and Practice* (Storch, J., Rodney, P. & Starzomski, R., eds), pp. 484–503. Pearson, Toronto.

Gadow, S. (1990) Existential advocacy. Philosophical foundations of nursing. In *Ethics in Nursing: An Anthology* (Pence, T. & Cantrall, J., eds), pp. 41–51. National League for Nursing, New York.

Levine, M. (1977) Nursing ethics and the ethical nurse. *American Journal of Nursing*, **77**(5): 846.

Watson, J. (1979) *Nursing: The Philosophy and Science of Caring*. Little Brown, Boston.

Watson, J. (1988) *Nursing: Human Science and Human Care, a Theory of Nursing*. National League for Nursing, New York.

Chapter 4

Reflective Practice and Socratic Dialogue

Gillian Todd

Reflective practice as a model for clinical supervision is a well established process in the training and professional development of nurse practitioners (Johns & Freshwater 1998; Rolfe *et al.* 2001). Although there is no universal agreement that defines reflective practice, Johns (1995, p. 2) captured the essence of the process: 'through reflection the practitioner may come to see the world differently, and based on these new insights may come to act differently as a changed person.'

The aims of reflective practice are ambitious in helping guide the supervisee through a process of learning and discovery. The supervisee learns to reflect-on-action through recalling and revisiting past events with an aim of learning from their experiences towards developing a new understanding of themselves and the situation. In time, through the process of clinical supervision, the reflective practitioner learns to reflect-in-action. This is the process whereby awareness of one's thoughts and actions is developed, allowing change in practice to take place (Schön 1983). One explanation for the shift from reflection-on-action to reflection-in-action could be the utilisation of the 'internal supervisor', which was first conceptualised by Casement (1985). Within the parameters of clinical supervision the development of the 'internal supervisor' is considered to be an advanced part of the reflective process (Bond & Holland 1998). The internal supervisor is a metaphor for Socratic dialogue that takes place within the reflective practitioner's consciousness in the moment, that allows spontaneous reflection-in-action to take place. The internal supervisor, through retrospective reflection-on-action on cognitive content and processes in clinical supervision, develops a meta-awareness of thoughts and associated behaviours. Glen *et al.* (1994) propose that the activation of critical self-consciousness fosters intellectual growth and behaviour change. The internal supervisor questions personal bias and subjectivity towards finding an objective perspective (Todd 2002). This process is often referred to as cognitive restructuring (Beck 1976; Beck *et al.* 1979). Laireiter & Willutzki (2003) consider self-reflection to be useful in helping the practitioner develop personal qualities and interpersonal competencies such as self-knowledge about blind spots, the development of a self-reflective working style and person-centred qualities of empathy and sensitivity. Reflection-in action is seen as an effective way of developing knowledge (Johns 1995; Jones

1995; Rolfe *et al.* 2001). Safran & Muran (2001) emphasise that the process of learning is experiential and not on a conceptual level. Clinical supervision provides a forum for experimentation and experiential learning. Fowler & Chevannes (1998) question the compatibility of reflection and clinical supervision in suggesting that for some people it may be unhelpful or even alien to their thinking style. Involving the self in being minimally defensive is considered to be a prerequisite for reflective practice.

As a clinical supervisor I have observed that supervisees engage with the process of guided reflection on different levels. Many nurse practitioners become reflective practitioners, and they attribute this to learning in clinical supervision. The experience of Mary, an intensive care nurse, captures this:

> "I feel I have progressed, so much more than I expected or how I expected. Having supervision with Gillian has given me a new depth to my role, work and life really. I truly feel that I have walked a path as such and come out of the other end richer."

However some supervisees do not develop with reflective practice alone and become very stuck.

Liz, an experienced community psychiatric nurse (CPN) engaged with clinical supervision, said she felt supported and that her work was validated. She would either bring 'success cases' or alternatively would say there was nothing to discuss because everything was fine. When I commented on my observation, Liz told me that because she was experienced she didn't always need help and that clinical supervision provided affirmation that she was a good nurse.

Although no advocate of reflective practice would claim it to be a panacea, I am left with a number of questions that challenge the assumptions of guided reflection (see Box 4.1) as a model for clinical supervision:

Box 4.1   Assumptions of guided reflection in clinical supervision

---

(1) The supervisee has the capacity to learn how to be a supervisee and can take responsibility for their role in clinical supervision.
(2) The supervisee has the capacity to be collaborative.
(3) The supervisee is a competent skilled technician.
(4) The subjective bias of retrospective reflection-on-action is the supervisee's reality in the present.
(5) The reflective practitioner has the ability to be open and honest in sharing thoughts, emotions and behaviour.
(6) The practitioner through reflection develops greater awareness of the self in relation to the self, others and the world.
(7) Developing meta-awareness of thoughts and self-defeating actions impacts on positive behaviour change.
(8) The practitioner has the capacity to develop multiple skills of reflection from reflection-on-action to reflection-in-action and reflect on content and process.
(9) The reflective practitioner develops a greater sense of knowing in which the process of reflection is integrated as part of the self.

(1) Do reflection-on-action and reflection-in-action bring about change in practice?
(2) If the practitioner develops a greater sense of knowing through reflection-on-action, what are the barriers to changing practice?
(3) Has the practitioner got the skills to change their practice?
(4) Is self-reflection selective reflection? What about what the supervisee isn't talking about?

Guided reflection, like all theories and models, has its limitations in assisting the reflective practitioner to develop both themselves and their practice. This chapter draws upon key principles from cognitive theories and therapy, and examines its application as an adjunct to guided reflection in clinical supervision.

Guided discovery

The theory and process of cognitive therapy are paralleled in cognitive therapy supervision (Padesky 1996).[1] There has been a growing interest in clinical supervision observational and outcome studies that have investigated the effects of multilevel clinical supervision involving systematically training clinical supervisors, the quality of clinical supervision, training the supervisee and associated patient outcome (Milne & James 2002; Milne *et al.* 2003). A number of small studies have analysed the components and structure of clinical supervision for cognitive therapy of which guided reflection is seen as central to the process of changing and improving clinical practice (Townsend *et al.* 2002; Bennett-Levy *et al.* 2003; Laireiter & Willutzki 2003). A number of themes from these studies have emerged:

(1) Embedded within the parallel process of cognitive therapy and cognitive therapy supervision is the supervisor's and supervisee's self-practice of cognitive therapy skills: in other words 'practising what we preach' (Bennett-Levy *et al.* 2003). In traditional schools of psychotherapy, for example humanistic and Freudian orientations, it would be mandatory for trainees to undergo personal therapy in order to develop the internal supervisor. What the cognitive therapists are alluding to is the development of their internal supervisor through self-reflection.
(2) Reflection-on-action takes place through case discussion.
(3) Interpersonal aspects of clinical supervision and the importance of the therapeutic alliance are central. The supervisor monitors the quality of the relationship with the supervisee (Safran & Muran 2001) and in turn models ways of addressing interpersonal impasses.
(4) Clinical supervision pays attention to the technical aspects through 'live' supervision strategies.

---

[1] A detailed description of cognitive theory and therapy can be found in Beck (1976, 1995); Beck *et al.* (1979); and Leahy & Dowd (2002).

Models of guided reflection assume technical skill and rely on the practitioner's description of their experience. I frequently ask myself: How do I know what the supervisee skills are? Is the reflective practitioner a scientist practitioner, in practising best practice based on best evidence? Is evidence based on acknowledging subjectivity good enough evidence? Has guided reflection in clinical supervision replaced the role of the lecturer/practitioner as the clinical supervisor who modelled nursing skills?

I would like to propose adding 'live' methods of clinical supervision based on cognitive therapy principles as an adjunct to guided reflection (see Box 4.2). However, there is a danger of being eclectic in this approach, which isn't my intention. Clinical supervision is a highly experiential process that is structured and collaborative. Padesky (1996, p. 271) believes that cognitive therapy employs guided discovery as an empirical investigative strategy, which is central to the primary learning process: 'Guided discovery is the engine that drives client learning.'

The terms 'guided discovery' and 'guided reflection' are interchangeable. Padesky & Greenberger (1995) described the key components of guided discovery as including a series of exploratory questions to uncover important information outside consciousness so as to enable accurate reflection and listening and the summarising and synthesising of the information discovered. Exploratory questions are most effectively asked using Socratic dialogue.[2] Wells (1997) considers that the aim of Socratic questioning is to explore the content and meaning of experiences to enable modification of cognition and behaviour. Wells suggests five basic requirements for effective Socratic questioning (Box 4.3).

In addition to general Socratic questions, Wells (1997) defines two other classes, the probe Socratic question and the reflective Socratic question. General Socratic questions are open-ended questions that aim to explore cognitions, emotions and behaviours, for example, 'In the situation how did you feel?' Probe Socratic questions aim to clarify issues and gain more detail, for example, 'What does feeling inadequate mean to you?' Reflective Socratic questions involve paraphrasing back the answers followed by another question, for example, 'When you felt uncertain and distressed, what were you thinking?'

Box 4.2 Live methods of clinical supervision as an adjunct to guided reflection

(1) Role play including modelling/demonstration of skills
(2) The use of audio/video recordings of clinical practice to promote reflection
(3) Live observation of practice
(4) The use of homework assignments in between clinical supervision sessions

---

[2] Socratic reflection and questioning originated from the Greek philosopher, Socrates. For examples of Socratic questions and the Socratic method, refer to the work of Overholser (1993a, 1993b).

Box 4.3   Essential components of Socratic questioning (adapted from Wells 1997)

(1)   The supervisor/therapist asks questions which the supervisee/client has the capacity to respond to.
(2)   The chosen questions focus on approaching a particular goal.
(3)   The questions aim to discover and explore new subject areas rather than close them down.
(4)   Questioning should not become an interrogation.
(5)   Reflected in the questions is genuine interest and curiosity about the supervisee's/client's experiences.

Padesky (1996) differentiates between the mode and focus of clinical supervision. The focus of clinical supervision refers to skills that the supervisee needs to develop, for example, guided reflection using Socratic questioning. The mode refers to the wide use of methods that will assist the supervisee in developing a range of skills necessary towards becoming a competent practitioner. Padesky considers a number of supervision principles. First, the supervisor builds on the supervisee's strengths, accurately commenting on the positive points. Through guided discovery and the use of Socratic questions the supervisee is encouraged to explore the weakness that will be the subsequent focus of clinical supervision sessions. The second principle is to use modes and foci of clinical supervision to build on the supervisee's strengths towards increasing clinical competence. Third, difficulties that the supervisee is experiencing need to be pinpointed in clinical supervision and worked through. The final principle is for the supervisor to pay attention to what isn't being discussed in clinical supervision. Socratic questioning is the vehicle by which these principles are applied. In the subsequent sections, methods of enhancing the development of the reflective practitioner through the use of Socratic dialogue and multiple 'live' methods of clinical supervision will be illustrated (see Box 4.3).

Role play

Role play can be used in a number of ways in clinical supervision to assist the supervisee in learning to be reflective. One way to use role play is as a demonstration of skill where the supervisor role-plays a situation with the supervisee as observer. The supervisee is asked to reflect-on-action guided by Socratic questioning. An example follows.

In supervision Sarah, a newly qualified ward nurse, reflected on a patient with whom she was working. She was having difficulty finding solutions to the patient's problems. Sarah was unsure how to try out new ways of approaching the problem with the patient. Socratic dialogue helped Sarah to generate a number of possibilities for how she might approach the problem. In a role-play dialogue Sarah re-enacted the role of her patient and the supervisor adopted the nurse practitioner role. The goal of the role play was to facilitate the exploration of emotions, thoughts and predictions that were pertinent to the situation. The supervisor and supervisee entered into a Socratic dialogue that drew upon the two classes of Socratic questions described by Wells (1997).

> *Supervisor*: "How did you feel in the role play [general Socratic question]?"
> *Supervisee*: "It was really interesting. I felt that I understood what my patient has been experiencing. My frustration with her disappeared. I felt warm towards her."
> *Supervisor*: "When you felt warm towards her, what thoughts went through your mind [reflective Socratic question]?"
> *Supervisee*: "I thought, 'When you're angry towards me it's because you're depressed and what's really happening is that you're angry with yourself.' I then remembered how much this patient is self-loathing to the point where she no longer cares for herself."
> *Supervisor*: "Role-playing your patient has given you empathy for her experiences [summary]. What observation did you make when I played the nurse practitioner role [probe Socratic question]?"
> *Supervisee*: "I noticed that you were very calm. You listened to me, which was demonstrated through the reflective phrases that you used. You made me feel valued and didn't leap in with telling me what I should be doing."
> *Supervisor*: "Having developed empathy for your patient and observed helpful ways of approaching the problem, what would you do differently [probe Socratic question]?"

Sarah uncovered and became aware of the strength of feeling and her communication style with the patient, of which she was previously unaware. Through developing empathy for the patient she was able to question her own reaction in relation to the patient.

The role play was reversed to enable Sarah to experiment with ways of approaching her patient, and this was again followed by Socratic dialogue.

Safran & Muran (2001, p. 13) observe: 'Role-playing various therapeutic responses in supervision should thus be viewed as a form of creative experimentation rather than learning a set of therapeutic responses through practice and rehearsal.' The supervisee as experimenter is invited to explore their thoughts and reactions, moving from reflection-on-action to reflection-in-action in the context of the safe environment of clinical supervision. Experiencing this process on an experiential level promotes self-awareness. The supervisee through personal discovery is encouraged to find their own inimitable solutions to the problem.

In addition to role play and reverse role play between two people, one person or a group can be involved in conducting role plays. Safran & Muran (2001) draw upon Gestalt therapy principles in suggesting self role plays. The supervisee plays two roles, the patient and the nurse practitioner. In order to heighten immersion in each role and to keep the roles distinct, two chairs are often used. The supervisor guides the supervisee through the process and might encourage the supervisee to respond as patient or nurse practitioner. The disadvantage of self role play can be that it is difficult to rapidly alternate between two roles. Nevertheless it is a very powerful strategy in promoting reflection.

In group clinical supervision a rolling chair role play can be used that involves the whole group participating. One supervisee role-plays the patient or their concern and in turn the other supervisees play the role of the nurse practitioner through Socratic dialogue to discover solutions and to develop self-awareness. The whole group is collaboratively using the forum of clinical supervision as a laboratory for experimentation and exploration.

The triadic role-play model is an interesting strategy for developing the internal supervisor. One supervisee role-plays the patient or their supervisory concern, the second supervisee is the nurse practitioner as clinical supervisor, and the third supervisee is an active external observer of the role-play situation. The observer offers technical advice and suggestions whilst in parallel becoming the inner voice of the internal supervisor. The nurse practitioner controls when to draw upon the advice of the observer who otherwise remains silent. A further role of the observer is to facilitate reflection-in-action in the clinical supervisor through the use of Socratic dialogue, which parallels the process between clinical supervisor and supervisee.

Role play is beyond doubt a powerful strategy for experiential learning in becoming a reflective practitioner, but it too has its limitations (see Box 4.4). It is worth noting that the supervisee needs to be carefully prepared for role-play situations. Any fears/reservations need to be elicited through engaging in Socratic dialogue itself.

Jane, a community psychiatric nurse working in elderly care, was adamant that she would not engage in a role-play situation. This created a barrier to clinical supervision. The following Socratic dialogue took place in clinical supervision:

Supervisor: "What is it about role play that you find difficult?"
Supervisee: "I'd just feel silly and probably make a fool of myself."
Supervisor: "What has been your experience of using role play in the past?"
Supervisee: "I've never done it before. I've always managed to avoid those situations."
Supervisor: "How do you know what a role play will actually be like if you've never tried it?"
Supervisee: "Well, I don't know I suppose."
Supervisor: "The disadvantages of role play are that you might feel silly and possibly make a fool of yourself. What do you think the advantages of role play might be?"
Supervisee: "I might learn something new about myself and learn new skills. If I discover that I'm not good at something, then it's better to know about it rather than hide from it. It will provide an opportunity to try out new ideas. I can't think of anything else right now."

Supervisor: "There's lots of good reasons to give it a go but we can't ignore your fear of been silly and making a fool of yourself. If this were a colleague in a similar situation, what would you say to her?"

Supervisee: "I'd say, 'What's the worse that could happen? No one has ever said that you are silly, so what reason would they have to be critical now? Just go for it.' "

Supervisor: "How convinced are you by what you would say to a colleague?"

Supervisee: "I'm very much convinced, I've just got to say that to myself."

Box 4.4   Advantages and disadvantages of role playing to promote self-reflection

Advantages of role play for the supervisee	Disadvantages of role play for the supervisee
(1) Re-enacting a situation as though it is happening in the present can help the supervisee make an accurate reinterpretation based on the experience. (2) The supervisee is encouraged to explore their thoughts, emotions and behaviour in relation to the supervision question. (3) Learning is experiential and does not rely on retrospective reflection. (4) Role play provides a canvas for creative experimentation with ideas. (5) It allows the development and practice of skills that are undeveloped in the supervisee. (6) Role play can be used to demonstrate 'best practice'.	(1) Role play can create discomfort and self-consciousness in some supervisees. (2) Supervisees might fear 'being exposed' as a bad nurse practitioner.
Advantages of role play for the supervisor	**Disadvantages of role play for the supervisor**
(1) The supervisor through observation is able to identify learning needs which have not previously been recognised. (2) The supervisor can assess the supervisee's capacity for reflection and the development of the internal supervisor. (3) The supervisor can learn from the supervisee.	(1) The supervisor assumes the role of expert in demonstrating skills with a danger of moving away from collaborative empiricism. (2) The supervisor might feel discomfort in exposing their strengths and weaknesses. The perfect role model is illusory, and learning often takes place when mistakes are made.

Audio/video recordings of clinical practice to promote reflection

The use of audio or video recordings of patient sessions, particularly in mental health nursing, is an important strategy in clinical supervision sessions for developing the reflective practitioner.[3] Padesky (1996, p. 283) considers the value of using audio/video material in clinical supervision:

> It is recommended that each supervision relationship include video, audio, or live observations of sessions because the supervisee's verbal summaries can describe, at best, only elements of the session within his or her current awareness and understanding. Observation of sessions alerts the supervisor to supervision needs that the supervisee might not recognise.

Critics of reflective practice would support Padesky's suggestion of using live supervision methods that can be objectively measured. One such is Hulatt (1995) who considered it preposterous that a 'sudden discovery' through reflection would develop a nurse's capacity for critical thought. Reflective practice has been condemned in the arena of quantitative research as lacking in scientific rigour. Common criticisms have been that 'its efficacy in improving outcome in patient care has not been demonstrated, and its lack of a scientific base provides methodological flaws in testing its validity' (Todd & Freshwater 1999, p. 1388). Ellis *et al.* (1996), after reviewing 144 empirical studies of clinical supervision, concluded that there was a lack of methodological and conceptual rigour. More recently, Milne *et al.* (2003, p. 193) argued that, in the field of mental health at least, clinical supervision was seen as important yet was a 'strikingly poorly researched topic'.

What is striking is the dichotomy of perceptions between two groups, the advocators of reflective practice who are mainly qualitative researchers (Johns & Freshwater 1998; Rolfe *et al.* 2001; Freshwater 2002), and the quantitative researchers who uphold the need for objectivity. Are we in fact singing the same song but using a different language? Are our goals for clinical supervision the same? A further factor, highlighted in Unger's (1996) study, was how the supervisory relationship was the most important factor related to outcome. Important factors that characterised the supervisory relationship were collaboration, trust, support and openness, along with allowing freedom and autonomy to the supervisee.

The use of video and audio illustrations of clinical practice as adjuncts to reflective practice allows the supervisee to self-observe their behaviour and through the process of reflection self-reinforce aspects of their nursing competencies. The nurse practitioner is also able to identify specific goals for

---

[3] When making tape/video recording, there are a number of ethical considerations. Written informed consent from the patient needs to be obtained. The patient should be informed as to the exact use of the tape, i.e. in supervision; how confidentiality will be maintained; and how the tapes will be stored; and it should be explained that the tape will be destroyed after an agreed period of time, i.e. after the supervision session.

self-development that can be achieved through clinical supervision. However, this strategy needs to be introduced within a reflective practice framework through the use of Socratic questioning.

There are Socratic questions that the supervisor could ask to elicit the supervisee's view of using audio/video recordings of clinical work to promote reflection:

- How do you feel about us using tape recordings of your clinical work in our supervision sessions [general Socratic question]?
- When you felt . . . , what thoughts ran through your mind [reflective Socratic question]?
- What are your reservations/concerns about listening to the tape [probe Socratic question]?
- What do you think are the benefits of listening to your tape [probe Socratic question]?

Through Socratic dialogue the supervisor elicits any concerns the supervisee might have about this procedure. Typical concerns include a fear of being exposed as a fraud, fear of negative evaluation by the supervisor, sounding/ looking foolish, can't bear hearing one's own voice, feeling self-conscious, audio/video recording will interfere with the therapeutic alliance, and patients will never agree to be audio/video recorded. Negative thoughts need to be challenged and tested out in supervision in order to help the supervisees view their concerns more realistically. The supervisor may choose to share recordings of their work to model open, non-defensive behaviour. This is based on the concept of parallel processes in the supervisor–supervisee/ supervisee–patient relationship.

There are three stages to using video/audio illustrations of clinical work.

(1) Preparing for the clinical supervision session. The supervisee needs to decide what they want the focus of the clinical supervision session to be. To help prepare for the clinical supervision session using audio/video information the supervisee should:
    - decide what concern/supervision question they want to explore
    - prioritise key concerns
    - decide how much time they need to allocate to each topic
    - prepare the segment of the tape/video they have decided to share
    - prepare a brief description of any relevant background information they think the supervisor should know to help explore their concern.
(2) Establish supervisee's and supervisor's guidelines for using audio/video review (see Box 4.5).
(3) Having reflected on the content of the audio/video material the third stage involves reflecting on processes involved using Socratic dialogue.

Ben, a CPN, shared a segment of his audio-taped recording of a counselling session with a depressed woman he was working with. He wanted to

Box 4.5   Guidelines for audio/video review in clinical supervision (adapted from Padesky 2002)

Supervisor guidelines	Supervisee guidelines
• Always start on a positive note. Make observations about two or three things that the supervisee is doing really well. • Observe one or two areas for improvement. • Notice your own reactions (thoughts, mood, behaviour, and physical reactions). Utilise your internal supervisor to question unhelpful reactions. • Ask the supervisee what area they would like to explore in clinical supervision. • Facilitate the reflective process through asking Socratic questions related to the video/audio illustration of clinical work. The video/audiotape can be paused at any moment to promote the reflective process. For example, 'What were you feeling at that moment?' 'What thoughts did you have?' 'What made you decide to do X?' 'What were you trying to achieve at that moment in time?' • Explore if the problem is recurrent (if so what are the maintaining factors?) or an isolated problem. • Ask the supervisee what they have learnt, and what they can do to implement new learning.	• View your clinical material through a positive lens first. Notice two to three things that you did well. • Notice your own reactions and reflect-in-action through utilising your internal supervisor. • Share your question/concern that you have decided to explore in clinical supervision. • Identify and reflect upon your thoughts and reactions to aspects of the tape that relate to your supervision question. • Reflect on the reasons why the problem is recurrent. • Decide in collaboration with your supervisor what areas of your practice have room for development and improvement. Select one or two areas to start with. • Ask yourself what you have learned through this experience. • How are you going to put this new knowledge into practice? • Identify times for practice (homework).

understand the reason why he felt frustrated and irritable with the patient. Initially Ben reflected-on-action using a reflective diary. He had tried to use his internal supervisor-in-action to try to understand his reactions but was feeling he had reached an impasse. We decided to stop the tape at a point where Ben was showing signs of irritability. We had the following dialogue:

Supervisor: "I want you to cast your mind back to the situation as if it were happening now. What are you feeling?"
Ben: "I'm feeling irritable, angry and very frustrated."
Supervisor: "Where in your body do you feel the emotion?"
Ben: "My neck and shoulders are tense and my stomach is churning."
Supervisor: "As you notice the tension in your neck, shoulders and stomach, what thoughts are going through your mind right now?"
Ben: "I can't stand this. You're pathetic."

Supervisor: "What do you mean by pathetic?"

Ben: "She's behaving in a helpless way, she won't do anything for herself and depends on other people all the time. I feel sorry for her husband and children having to live with such a miserable woman. Every time I make suggestions, she ignores my advice and chooses to wallow in self-pity. I'm feeling wound up now just saying that. I'd no idea that I felt so strongly."

Supervisor: "How do you feel about yourself when your patient ignores your advice?"

Ben: "I think that I have failed her, failed as a CPN, and consequently I feel hopeless."

Supervisor: "What impact do you think your negative interpretation of your work as a CPN has upon your relationship with your patient?"

Ben: "I lose empathy and start blaming her for how I'm feeling about myself, which in turn isn't helping her. She already feels rejected by others and covertly I am adding to her distress."

Supervisor: "What do you need to work on before your next meeting with the patient?"

Ben: "I need to practise dealing with my own emotional reactions to re-establish a good therapeutic alliance. I need to remind myself of the nature of depression and try to understand her experience."

Live observation of practice

Direct observation of clinical practice can be immensely helpful in identifying supervision needs to enhance the process of developing as a skilled nurse and reflective practitioner. The development of technical skills needs to develop in parallel with skills of reflection and cannot be separated. In my training as a clinical supervisor, each training session would include learning about the theoretical aspects of clinical supervision and a practical session in which experiential learning took place. The classroom became a laboratory for experimentation. In a small group setting each nurse practitioner had the opportunity to practise and test out being both the supervisee and the supervisor. The group observed the supervision session from three different lenses, the content of the dialogue, the process of supervision including fidelity to the model of reflective practice and the supervisor's ability to conceptualise the supervisee's issues. At the end of the observed session both supervisor and supervisee were asked to reflect through the use of Socratic dialogue on their experience. This involved identifying what went well and also what areas needed further work. The group then gave accurate feedback to the supervisor, again starting on a positive note followed by suggestions for future improvement. Reflecting on my roles as supervisee, supervisor and observer of supervisor and supervisee allowed me to view and experience the practice of reflection from multiple angles, thereby helping me develop empathy and a greater understanding of the processes involved.

The next stage of training involves supervising nurses in our areas of work that involves transferring the newly learnt skills from one area to another. The parallel relationships are supervisor–supervisor, supervisor–supervisee and supervisee–patient. I have shared this experience in supervising my supervisees through encouraging live observation of their practice. One reason for my decision to include live observation stemmed from consideration of the point made by Bond & Holland (1998). They noticed that mental health nurses were prone to overestimate their ability to reflect in clinical supervision and demonstrated a tendency to make inappropriate and often dangerous psychotherapy interventions that pathologised aspects of nursing practice. Consequently, good interpersonal skills such as active listening were reduced. One explanation for the exaggeration of the nurses' capacity to reflect could be that mental health nurses tend to equate experience with skill. How do you know that the experience is a good experience? How can you judge what learning if any has taken place as a consequence of that experience?

Introducing the idea of live observation can be a delicate matter that can provoke considerable anxiety and fear of negative evaluation. There are three main modes of live observation, these being:

(1) Supervisor observing the supervisee like a member of an audience, distant and not involved in the clinical area.
(2) Supervisor viewing the supervisee through a one-way mirror or video link.
(3) Supervisor and supervisee working as co-therapists.

The supervisor needs to match the mode of live observation to the supervision goal, for example learning to reflect-in-action in conceptualising the patient's problems. At the end of a live observation session the supervisor and supervisee also need to reflect on the process, once again using Socratic dialogue (see Box 4.6).

Box 4.6   Socratic questions to facilitate the process of reflection-on-action following live observation of clinical practice

Session content and session process
• What do you think went well in the session?
• What have you learnt (prompts: about yourself/the patient/therapeutic relationship/ skills)?
• What did you find difficult?
• How might you have done things differently?
• What areas do you need to work on?
• How do you plan to do this?

The use of homework assignments

Homework is an integral, not optional, part of clinical supervision in helping the nurse practitioner develop higher order skills of reflection. In drawing a parallel with psychotherapy, Neimeyer & Feixas (1990) found that patients who completed homework assignments as part of group cognitive therapy made more progress in developing skill and knowledge compared with those patients who didn't complete homework. What is the purpose of introducing in-between clinical supervision session homework? Clinical supervision sessions typically last 1 hour and for most practitioners occur once or twice a month during which most nurses have spent between 75 and 150 hours engaged in clinical practice. It is crucial that practice in self-supervision take place to a model to refine the development of the internal supervisor (the inner voice of reflection-in-action) in addition to practising and developing clinical skills. Bennett-Levy *et al.* (2003) believe the key component in the development of therapeutic competence is achieved through continuous professional reflection. In Box 4.7 I outline some of the variety of modes of homework in clinical supervision.

Box 4.7   Modes of homework in clinical supervision to enhance reflexivity

---
(1)   Keeping a reflective journal for reflection-on-action
(2)   Observing audio/video recordings of own work to practice self-reflection
(3)   Becoming aware of thoughts, emotions and actions in the clinical setting
(4)   Practising reflecting-in-action whilst simultaneously attending to the situation
(5)   Reading material to increase knowledge

When considering setting homework a number of principles apply. Homework needs to be tailored to the individual's needs and to be decided upon collaboratively. It needs to be established as a win–win situation, so the supervisee must have the level of skill to accomplish what is being asked of them. This is an important aspect of promoting development and learning and enables the experience to have a positive outcome. A final consideration is the need to examine the time and resources available in which to complete homework and to identify any potential barriers.

Emma, a trainee clinical supervisor, was a participant in a reflexive case study research project that investigated the processes involved in developing the internal supervisor. For homework we both agreed to keep a reflective journal and to listen to a tape recording of the sixth clinical supervision session. Box 4.8 provides extracts from our reflective diaries. Part 1 illustrates reflections on reflexive writing, and in part 2 extracts from reflections on listening to the audio recordings are presented.

Box 4.8   Extracts from the reflective diaries

Part 1: Maintaining a reflective journal and reflexive writing

Extracts from my reflective journal (clinical supervisor)
This was the first time that I had regularly kept a reflective journal mainly because I considered myself to be reflective and failed to see any value in writing my thoughts down, but I was wrong in assuming so. Recording my reflections-on-action on paper helped me to learn skills of reflection-in-action.

Extracts from Emma's reflective journal (supervisee)
Once I started writing it just flowed; it went right on to paper. As I reflected on one thing it led to another. I couldn't get the words down quick enough. I chose Rolfe's reflexive journal format as my diary: reading your reflections then reflecting on what you have written takes you to a deeper level of reflection.

Part 2: Tape recording the clinical supervision session

Extracts from my reflective journal (clinical supervisor)
As I listened to the tape I noticed my hesitation in helping Emma explore her critical incident and wondered what was holding me back. At one point I was speechless, which made me question the issue of transference. Emma's distress had become mine, rendering me ineffective for that moment. I had taken on the role of Atlas, feeling the burden and pressures of the world. Although the supervision session had passed and could not be changed, my internal supervisor was reflecting-in-action on the process of listening to the tape. Replaying the session is helpful insofar as I can be more objective in my reflection-on-action that shapes and modifies my internal supervisor. I wonder if there are parallels in reflecting-on-action from memory after the clinical encounter and with reflecting-on-action whilst listening to the tape?

Extracts from Emma's reflective journal (supervisee)
When I listened to the tape I did not realise how much I reflect. Listening to myself helped me reflect about my reflections and I was able to give myself credit for my achievement in consciously becoming a reflective practitioner. It is my ability to be reflective that makes me a good nurse. How can I take this further?

Concluding thoughts

I have suggested a number of adjunct principles borrowed and expanded from cognitive behavioural theories and therapy. As I have argued, guided reflection, as with all models and theories, is of limited value when applied in a concrete and linear manner (see Chapter 1 for further elaboration on this point). Drawing upon the concept of Socratic dialogue and utilising cognitive behavioural techniques, I invite the practitioner and supervisor to broaden their options with regard to the modalities for facilitating and guiding reflection on practice.

References

Beck, A.T. (1976) *Cognitive Therapy and the Emotional Disorders*. Penguin Books, Harmondsworth.

Beck, A.T., Rush, J.A., Shaw, B.F. and Emery, G. (1979) *Cognitive Therapy of Depression*. Guilford, New York.

Beck, J. (1995) *Cognitive Therapy: Basics and Beyond*. Guilford Press, New York.

Bennett-Levy, J., Lee, N., Travers, K., Pohlman, S. and Hamernik, E. (2003) Cognitive therapy from inside out: enhancing therapist skills through practising what we preach. *Behavioural and Cognitive Psychotherapy*, **31**(2): 143–58.

Bond, M. and Holland, S. (1998) *Skills of Clinical Supervision for Nurses*. Open University Press, Buckingham.

Casement, P. (1985) *On Learning from the Patient*. Guilford Press, New York.

Ellis, M.V., Ladany, N., Krengel, M. and Schuldt, D. (1996) Clinical supervision research from 1981 to 1993: a methodological critique. *Journal of Counselling Psychology*, **43**: 35–50.

Fowler, J. and Chevannes, M. (1998) Evaluating the efficacy of reflective practice within the context of clinical supervision. *Journal of Advanced Nursing*, **27**: 379–82.

Freshwater, D. (ed.) (2002) *Therapeutic Nursing: Improving Patient Care through Reflection*. Sage, London.

Glen, S., Clark, A. and Nicol, M. (1994) Reflecting on reflection: a personal encounter. *Nurse Education Today*, **15**(2): 61–8.

Hulatt, I. (1995) A sad reflection. *Nursing Standard*, **9**(20): 22–3.

Johns, C. (1995) The value of reflective practice for nursing. *Journal of Clinical Nursing*, **4**(1): 23–30.

Johns, C. and Freshwater, D. (1998) *Transforming Nursing through Reflective Practice*. Blackwell Science, Oxford.

Jones, P.R. (1995) Hindsight bias in reflective practice: an empirical investigation. *Journal of Advanced Nursing*, **21**(4): 783–8.

Laireiter, A.R. and Willutzki, U. (2003) Self-reflection and self-practice in training of cognitive behaviour therapy: an overview. *Clinical Psychology and Psychotherapy*, **10**(1): 19–30.

Leahy, R.L. and Dowd, T.E. (eds) (2002) *Clinical Advances in Cognitive Psychotherapy*. Springer, New York.

Milne, D.L. and James, I.A. (2002) The observed impact of training on competence in clinical supervision. *British Journal of Clinical Psychology*, **41**: 55–72.

Milne, D.L., Pilkington, J., Gracie, J. and James, I. (2003) Transferring skills from supervision to therapy: a qualitative and quantitative N = 1 analysis. *Behavioural and Cognitive Psychotherapy*, **31**(2): 193–202.

Neiemeyer, R.A. and Feixas, G. (1990) The role of homework and skill acquisition in the outcome of group cognitive therapy for depression. *Behavior Therapy*, **21**(3): 281–92.

Overholser, J.C. (1993a) Elements of the Socratic method: I Systematic questioning. *Psychotherapy*, **30**: 67–74.

Overholser, J.C. (1993b) Elements of the Socratic method: II Inductive reasoning. *Psychotherapy*, **30**: 75–85.

Padesky, C.A. (1996) Developing cognitive therapist competency: teaching and supervision models. In *Frontiers of Cognitive Therapy* (Salkovskis, P.M., ed.), pp. 226–92. Guilford, New York.

Padesky, C.A. and Greenberger, D. (1995) *Clinician's Guide to Mind over Mood*. Guilford Press, New York.

Rolfe, G., Freshwater, D. and Jasper, M. (2001) *Critical Reflection for Nurses and the Caring Professions: A User's Guide*. Palgrave, Basingstoke.

Safran, J.D. and Muran, C.J. (2001) A relational approach to training and supervision in cognitive psychotherapy. *Journal of Cognitive Psychotherapy*, **15**(1): 3–15.

Schön, D.A. (1983) *The Reflective Practitioner*. Basic Books, London.

Todd, G. (2002) The role of the internal supervisor in developing therapeutic nursing. In *Therapeutic Nursing* (Freshwater, D., ed.), pp. 58–82. Sage, London.

Todd, G., and Freshwater, D. (1999) Reflective practice and guided discovery: clinical supervision. *British Journal of Nursing*, **8**(20): 1383–9.

Townsend, M., Iannetta, L. and Freeston, M.H. (2002) Clinical supervision in practice: a survey of UK cognitive behavioural psychotherapists accredited by the BABCP. *Behavioural and Cognitive Psychotherapy*, **30**(4): 485–500.

Unger, D.B. (1996) Core problems in clinical supervision: factors related to outcome. Unpublished dissertation. California School of Professional Psychology, Berkeley.

Wells, A. (1997) *Cognitive Therapy for Anxiety Disorder*. Wiley, New York.

Chapter 5

Clinical Supervision in the Context of Custodial Care

Dawn Freshwater

Today the surveillance screen tends to replace the window.

(Virilio 1996)

The term 'clinical supervision' originates in the training and practice of counselling and psychotherapy. However, whilst supervision has been an integral part of counselling and psychotherapy for many years, it is only relatively recently that more formal structures for monitoring its implementation and effectiveness have been put into place through such bodies as the United Kingdom Council for Psychotherapy and the British Association for Counselling. Many of the functions of therapy and counselling have parallels with nursing and other health-related disciplines. The notion of the caring relationship and a therapeutic alliance is fundamental not only to psychotherapy but also to nursing, and there are similar requirements for self-awareness and interpersonal and emotional coping skills for nurses as there are for therapists (Briant & Freshwater 1998; Freshwater 2002, 2003). Swain (1995), for example, suggests that clinical supervision could provide nursing with a containing and holding environment comparable to that of Winnicott's (1991) facilitating environment. A number of developments in nursing (including the Allitt inquiry and the subsequent Clothier report) have led to the publication of several position statements regarding the implementation of clinical supervision into nursing (see, for example, UKCC 1996). However, the discourse around clinical supervision and its relationship to reflective practice has created an interesting and sometimes polarised debate within the literature (Fowler & Chevannes 1999; Heath & Freshwater 2000; Cotton 2001; Gilbert 2001). As an experienced therapist with a background in nursing and health care I have been involved in and contributed to the development of this discourse over a number of years, primarily as a supervisor, but also as a researcher and trainer. The focus of this chapter is my own reflection on the notion of reflection and clinical supervision as confessional practices within the context of surveillance. In order to facilitate discussion I will refer to a number of practice development and research initiatives involving the implementation of clinical supervision within a prison health care environment.

The majority of nurses working in prisons are qualified nurses who, on a daily basis, are dealing with deeply disturbed individuals manifesting their emotional, psychological and spiritual distress through polarisation and splitting of feelings, self and other. Aggression, paranoia and fear are pervasive, with many inmates swinging between violence against others and self-harm. Many of the staff are working both as therapists and nurses, coping with the patients' physical needs as well as other sources of distress; most have some training in counselling; few, however, have access to clinical supervision (Freshwater *et al.* 2001, 2002; see also Chapter 6 in this book). Those who do have access find it difficult to engage in supervision. Drawing upon my previous works I will be referring to specific theoretical and practical learning. I will be attending to this low level of acceptance of clinical supervision within the prison health care system, and will describe the approaches taken as a result of this, drawing directly upon clinical experience to outline the implications for the supervisory alliance of working within a custodial environment.

Recent developments in health care have seen nursing practice assigned the task of implementing clinical supervision and evidence-based practice (UKCC 1996). There has been and continues to be widespread confusion about the nature and purpose of clinical supervision in health care settings following the publication of a position paper on clinical supervision by the United Kingdom Central Council for Nurses, Midwives and Health Visitors in 1996 (UKCC 1996). The confusion exists, to some extent, as a result of the very different views that are espoused both within the literature and across disciplines. Some NHS trusts have interpreted clinical supervision as managerial and hierarchical, whilst individual bodies continue with previously adopted approaches. Midwives and social workers, for example, have been involved in managerial supervision for several decades. However, the culture of nursing is different. Having experienced years of oppression and subservience, the notion of managerial/hierarchical supervision is met with distrust, antagonism and resistance. So, although it is unlikely that there are now many nurses who have not heard about clinical supervision, its implementation remains patchy and lacks a systematic strategy, with poor use of models and a clear lack of reflection (Bishop & Freshwater 2000; Rolfe *et al.* 2001). Despite this, little has been done to encourage individual ownership at local level through education, needs analyses and supportive interventions.

To date, then, in many areas clinical supervision is viewed by those in the caring professions (although certainly not entirely) as being linked to surveillance, and as such has been received with little enthusiasm. This notion of surveillance is of particular relevance not only to the context of supervision in health care, but also to the prison service.

Nursing in secure environments

In 1999 the UKCC published the findings of a project entitled 'Nursing in secure environments'. The report reached a number of conclusions and recommendations related to the lack of formal systems of professional support and mentorship available to those nurses who are working in conditions that test their professional resilience. Two of the main points were highlighted as a result of the project. First, the implementation of clinical supervision for nursing and related staff (prison health care officers) was inconsistent; and second, there was a major tension in the practice of those staff between the need for clinical supervision and the lack of understanding, resources (in terms of time and expertise) and the subsequent lack of investment in professional development. This continues to present a challenge given that paragraph 59 of the prison nurses report (NHSE 2000) recommends that all staff working in a nursing capacity should have regular clinical supervision:

> The possibility of accessing support and supervision outside the prison should be explored, particularly in smaller establishments. (The term 'professional supervision' is used here to mean the opportunity to review and reflect on practice and performance, critical incidents and achievements.)

> (NHSE 2000, p. 24)

For further analysis and an historical overview of this work I refer the reader to Chapter 6. For now I will concentrate on the issue of professional self-regulation, relating this to reflective practice and the concept of surveillance.

Professional self-regulation versus surveillance – the normative function of supervision?

The profession of nursing is predominantly self-regulatory. Practitioners are guided by a code of conduct and codes of ethics that act as rules that serve to uphold the safety of the patient, whether they are a sick person in a hospital bed or a client who has chosen to enter therapy to examine their personal life experiences (UKCC 1992). The codes of conduct espouse a number of rules that to a certain extent govern the behaviour of the individual practitioner, supervisor and trainer, and the larger group or profession; a number of reciprocal rewards and punishments are put in place, for example registration. Supervision is one method of monitoring the effectiveness of the codes of conduct and ethics and regulating the minimum standard both of individual practice and of education and training organisations (Proctor 1986). One of the effects of surveillance is to make the person effectively self-regulatory, that is, an autonomous practitioner. Gilbert (2001, p. 200) is sceptical of the concept of an autonomous practitioner, particularly when linked to the notion of a self-management model such as that espoused within reflective practice and clinical supervision. He argues that:

> the identification of individual nurses as autonomous practitioners brings with it a moral superiority that can become symbolised through accredited roles such as 'clinical supervisor' or 'advanced nurse practitioner'.

As Gilbert (2001, p. 202) is at great pains to explain, 'Clinical supervision and reflective practice make individual practitioners "visible" and through this visibility subject to modes of surveillance.' There is little doubt that such self-regulatory practices as reflective practice (and guided reflection through supervision) do have the gentle touch of surveillance in the Foucauldian (Foucault 1980) sense. The concept of surveillance is epitomised by the invention of Bentham's panopticon, a circular prison which accommodates the prisoners in cells around the periphery. In this way they can all be observed by a single guard placed in the centre. As Burr & Butt (2000, p. 190) comment:

> The panopticon's efficiency and innovation is that prisoners – who live with the constant knowledge that their behaviour might at any moment be scrutinised – come to internalise the 'gaze' of the guard and thus incorporate this monitoring and control into their own selves.

The notion of an internalised gaze is comparable to that of Casement's (1985) internal supervisor. However, as in any other relationship that has a power imbalance (patient/therapist; nurse/patient; prison officer/inmate; supervisor/supervisee), the face of the internalised gaze can take on any number of expressions, from attacking and punitive to one of support and encouragement.

Gilbert (2001), and also Cotton (2001), who draws upon the Orwellian (1989) idea of the thought police in her analysis of reflective practice, point out that regulation of the population is a feature not just of prisons but of all institutions and organisations which control members though hierarchies, divisions and norms – including, of course, nursing and the health professions. Parker (1999), for example, in his deconstruction of psychotherapy, discusses the possibility of psychotherapy as a normalising practice, which has implications for the process of supervision and its own role in normalising the practice of psychotherapy itself. Psychotherapy, he argues, presumes to bring about a restructuring or reprogramming of behaviour against some socially acceptable criterion of the normal, the deviant, the well adjusted and so on. In this way psychotherapy can be viewed as a political and social activity, serving the community and potentially reinforcing (maybe even defining) what is socially acceptable and what is deviant. In the same way Gilbert (2001) argues that supervision parallels this process, just as some theoretical models depend upon the concept of the parallel process within the client/therapist–supervisee/supervisor relationships. Supervision, it could be argued, monitors the level of deviance in the counsellor and psychotherapist against normative criteria as defined in the code of ethics and practice (there is, of course, one for supervisors too). Similarly, in nursing, it could be posited that reflection guided through clinical supervision monitors the level of deviance from protocols, codes of conduct and policies, this through a confessional practice. This, in itself, is an interesting point to debate: whilst this might be one aspect of clinical supervision, it is just that, *one* aspect, that for many is background rather than foreground. Nevertheless, it is a significant backdrop, affecting the relationship, the contract, the dynamic and the energy within the alliance.

But what of reflection and supervision that take place within a social system which has deviance as its norm, which relies upon the external gaze of society for its existence and upon its internalised gaze for survival?

The neurotic gaze: the panoptical model of clinical supervision

Reggie and Ronnie Kray, two of the world's most famous criminals, discuss their coping strategies for surviving in a prison environment in their book *Our Story* (Kray & Kray 1988). Cohen and Taylor (1992), in the sociological research report *Escape Attempts*, are other examples of writers describing what equates to early psychodynamic (schizoid) defence mechanisms such as projection and splitting (Klein 1975). Others are objectified, with the I–it relationship dominating (Buber 1958). It is interesting to note that this way of being is also adopted by the staff working within health care systems as they struggle with their own vulnerabilities and to maintain their own safety (Menzies-Lyth 1988; Briant & Freshwater 1998). There are splits that operate within the prisons themselves, with the hospital wing (and the nurses) being viewed as a 'haven' by the inmates. For those inmates experiencing persecution (of both an internal and an external nature), self-harm is one way of achieving a period of 'letting go', being held safe in the arms of mother/nurse. For some, trust is not an option: there is no escaping the paranoia; it travels with them into the hospital wing and the nursing staff take on the role of good and bad mother (albeit unconsciously).

The prison nursing staff are not, however, without their own persecutory complexes, as is seen, for example, in the paranoia regarding the implementation of guided reflection through supervision. A recent research study involved my developing group supervision within the prison health care system following some basic training in the role and function of clinical supervision (see Chapter 6). On further discussion with the staff in one prison during training, it was revealed that much of the paranoia around clinical supervision related to confidentiality and trust, specifically regarding what the 'stories' told in supervision would be used for. Gilbert (2001) argues that such practices as clinical supervision are confessional in that they incite staff, through 'speech or writing', to 'reveal the truth about themselves'. It would appear that many practitioners within the prison environment were particularly paranoid about what would happen to their 'confessions' or truths – that is, once private thoughts were expressed in a public sphere.

In exploring the suspiciousness of the staff in more depth, it was unsurprising to discover that it was not just active within the prison walls. The lack of trust and subsequent suspicion were a part of the practitioner's everyday life. Some post-modern writers are beginning to articulate the maladies of our contemporary lifestyles and note this sense of pervasive 'reasonable suspicion' experienced by the practitioners:

When everyday life increasingly unfolds in institutions which are obsessed by the need to observe, by a fetish for more information, and by the tacit assumption that everyone is suspect, we should perhaps accept the notion that entire social systems can be paranoid. In such a situation, individual diagnoses become farcical.

(Fee 2000, p. 32)

As Fee observes, our current social climate makes it difficult to be clear about boundaries, what belongs to whom, and whom to trust. I believe this is amplified in the prison environment, which houses those people who carry society's shadow. In addition, those employees of the prison service are dealing with the projections of both inmates and media, as well as casting out their own shadow for projection. This is also part of the 'bigger picture' or 'collective', for, as Johnson (1991, p. 26) says:

To refuse the dark side of one's nature is to store up or accumulate darkness . . . We are presently dealing with the accumulation of a whole society that has worshipped its light side and refused the dark . . .

It has been interesting to explore the implementation of clinical supervision within the context of custodial care where paranoia and lack of trust are constant companions for staff and inmates alike. Challenges that are presented include how to work with staff whose primitive defences are foreground and who are coping not only with the projections and splitting of the prisoners but also often with their own and others' unconscious ones. It is paradoxical that an environment that provides literal and rigid boundaries is not felt to be a safe container. How can a supervisor support the development of a safe container within an environment that is so closely linked to the panopticon, without supervision becoming the experience of the panopticon itself? It could be argued, however, that the panoptical model of clinical supervision, with the supervisor in the position of voyeur, may have something to contribute to the debate.

Voyeurism and the shadow – a reflection

Reflecting upon the notion of supervision as self-regulation, I wish to pause at this point to notice the fascination that this work has held for me, not only as a therapist, supervisor and nurse, but also (and more importantly) as a person. Criminality is fascinating, as Cohen and Taylor (1992, p. 32) observe:

we were as interested as anyone else in finding out what famous criminals really looked like, in comparing their 'underworld' stereotypes with their actual behaviour . . . we justified the talk, however, by reference to our criminological interests.

I have discovered my own curiosity and desire for deviance, my surprise at the pleasure that is derived from witnessing the destructive instinct (*Thanatos* in action) and the powerful energy that is behind fantasies and imaginations fuelled by hermetic tales of half truths, distortions, and unexpected twists and turns. I have found that my need for supervision of supervision (i.e. self-regulation) has increased as I notice my desire to find out more about the details of crimes committed when supervisees present their client. Unsure whether I am being drawn off the scent, or if this is the scent, I am aware of my wonderings. I have met 'known' murderers and 'paedophiles', who appear to me to be like many other distressed individuals attempting to make meaning out of their experiences. And I have worked with staff who are trying to make meaning out of their experience of being with these individuals and their own lives. My reflections lead me to believe that we are all potential (and to a limit, actual) criminals: one of the differences between someone who carries out a murder and myself is self-regulation and ethical watchfulness, that is, a certain type of surveillance. This leads me to question whether there isn't a contextual typology of surveillance, within which surveillance and confessional practices consist of different qualities. To refer back to Gilbert (2001), it is of course important to be 'visible' and thus accountable in one's professional practice, as well as within one's day-to-day life. I believe that where both he and I agree is that all such practices necessitate a degree of deconstruction and reflexivity, both by those authors who espouse such models, and importantly by those practitioners engaged in the practical processes. However, not all practitioners will either be capable of, or indeed want to, reflect at that level.

Implications for the supervisory alliance

Page and Woskett (1994) describe the first phase of their model as contracting. There are a number of components to this phase which serve to guide the supervisory alliance. As previously mentioned, one of the key concerns of the prison nursing staff in embarking upon clinical supervision was that of confidentiality, which closely linked with the wish for non-hierarchical and non-managerial supervision. Following a basic training in supervision, all staff were given the opportunity to take up voluntary supervision. Supervisees were given both information about the purpose and functions of clinical supervision (including formative, educative and supportive functions: Proctor 1986) and the ethical mapping model (Johns & Freshwater 1998).

They were also asked to reflect on their own beliefs, values and opinions. All groups (five in total) were encouraged to devise their own ground rules, including their expectations of each other and of myself as facilitator. None of this was entirely new to the groups as many had completed some form of basic counselling skills course; only one art therapist was already in supervision and proved to be a valuable asset to the training course. Questions were regularly raised regarding the issues of confidentiality, safety and trust, and, as already mentioned, parallels were drawn with the client group. One supervisee reflected on the fact that it was difficult to trust anyone else unless she could trust herself, something she had been questioning since joining the prison service. It was decided that confidentiality could never be absolute; the aim of the ground rules therefore was to establish the limits of confidentiality.

As the supervisor my initial aim has been to establish boundaries which are representative of a safe container. Whilst there are strong and rigid boundaries in prisons, they are not necessarily perceived as creating safety, unless you are on the outside of them. I was torn in the beginning about including my own fears and anxieties and the notion of creating safety. I knew I needed to include my fear of the prison, of being locked in, of depending on others for my own safety, but wanted to do this in a permissive way, whilst being aware of also being the supervisory role model. In the first session of supervision in one prison, I encouraged the whole group to meditate on the part of them that wanted to be there and the part of them that did not. The group members voiced my fears; they talked of their own fear, of having to 'trust' others to maintain a safe environment and the pressure they felt under to 'hold things together'. For one supervisee, the part of her that did not want to be there was the part that might not hold it together. We used the metaphor of the 'locked door' to imagine what was being held back, locked away, kept safe, and I referred to the story of Bluebeard.

Within the space that was created by the structure of clinical supervision I was functioning at many levels: as supervisor, group member, outsider, insider, etc. As a group facilitator I was also aware of the group as an intrapersonal group (with the focus on the process within the individual). This can best be described as individual supervision with an audience. My awareness of this particular approach being a bit like eavesdropping and its potential for buying into persecutory feelings has meant that I erred on the side of affirming/nurturing supervisor. At the interpersonal level (with the focus on what happens between individuals), I was consciously aware of making use of the other members of the group as a resource, building on skills that already existed as a result of previous counselling training and experience. The group examined parallel processes and patterns that manifest between themselves as a group, as a staff group and across other sectors of the prison.

The groups were and were not functioning at the transpersonal level group (that is looking beyond the individual). They were not well enough established to be able to (consciously) view the group as being more than simply the sum of the intrapersonal and interpersonal events. However, as they have become more of a working group, the staff are more aware of their defences and the symbolism that the prison holds for the psyche, they feel less threatened and they reveal more of their soulfulness.

Space has been made for archetypes, goddesses, gods, the shadow and oscillation between the literal and symbolic assist with the balance between challenge and support. Space has been made for guilt, sadness, longing and repulsion. Affirmation has been given to staff who suffer angst about their obvious favouritism, and Oedipus has journeyed heroically alongside those nurses who find themselves rescuing. Tears have been cried both in despair and in black humour. Thus one supervisee related her experience of finding her patient in the toilet trying to strangle himself by having string around his neck attached to his shoe so that as he put his foot to the ground he could not breathe. As she lifted his leg high above his head, he screamed in pain, saying, 'Stop! That hurts!'

Many of the inmates have pictures on the walls of the cells. The staff have now decided to adorn their own clinical supervision room with poetry books and art. The room is increasingly used for 'quiet time', for periods of self-surveillance and for observing the internal gaze.

The notion of containment in a facilitating custodial environment may seem like an oxymoron. Containment, however, is at the heart of 'custodial care'. Nevertheless, it presents a challenge for supervisor, supervisee and inmate. Where there is containment, there is the transpersonal. The longing that I have witnessed (and experienced) during my development as a supervisor within the prison health care system suggests that the transpersonal is not only seeking but being sought.

My walk through prison gardens, the rituals observed in caring for personal possessions and my tour of prison art blocks spoke to me of the soul of the inmates. My privileged position as witness to the nurses' experiences confirmed the existence of transpersonal aspects of humanity deeply embedded in everyday practice.

References

Bishop, V. and Freshwater, D. (2000) Report on a multi-site, multidisciplinary evaluation of clinical supervision. De Montfort University, Leicester.

Briant, S. and Freshwater, D. (1998) Exploring mutuality within the nurse–patient relationship. *British Journal of Nursing*, **7**(4): 204–11.

Buber, M. (1958) *I and Thou*. Scribner, New York.

Burr, V. and Butt, T. (2000) *Psychological Distress and Post-modern Thought*. Sage, London.

Casement, P. (1985) *On Learning from the Patient*. Routledge, London.

Cohen, S. and Taylor, L. (1992) *Escape Attempts*. Routledge, London.

Cotton, A.H. (2001) Private thoughts in public spheres: issues of reflection and reflective practices in nursing. *Journal of Advanced Nursing*, **36**(4): 512–19.

Fee, D. (2000) (ed.) *Pathology and the Post-modern*. Sage, London.

Foucault, M. (1980) *The Confession of the Flesh. Power/Knowledge. Selected interviews and other writings, 1972–1977*. Harvester, Wiltshire.

Fowler, J. and Chevannes, M. (1999) Evaluating the efficacy of reflective practice within the context of clinical supervision. *Journal of Advanced Nursing*, **27**(2): 379–82.

Freshwater, D. (2002) *Therapeutic Nursing: Improving Patient Care through Reflection*. Sage, London.

Freshwater, D. (2003) *Counselling Skills for Nurses, Midwives and Health Visitors*. Open University Press, Buckingham.

Freshwater, D., Storey, L. and Walsh, L. (2001) Developing leadership through clinical supervision: part one. *Nursing Management*, **8**(8): 10–13.

Freshwater, D., Walsh, L. and Storey, L. (2002) Developing leadership through clinical supervision: part two. *Nursing Management*, **8**(9): 16–20.

Gilbert, T. (2001) Reflective practice and clinical supervision: meticulous rituals of the confession. *Journal of Advanced Nursing*, **36**(2): 199–205.

Heath, H. and Freshwater, D. (2000) Clinical supervision as an emancipatory process: avoiding inappropriate intent. *Journal of Advanced Nursing*, **32**(5): 1298–306.

Johns, C. and Freshwater, D. (1998) *Transforming Nursing through Reflective Practice*. Blackwell Science, Oxford.

Johnson, R.A. (1991) *Owning Your Own Shadow*. Harper, San Francisco.

Klein, M. (1975) *The Writings of Melanie Klein*, Vol. 3. Hogarth, London.

Kray, R. and Kray, R. (1988) *Our Story*. Sidgwick and Jackson, London.

Menzies-Lyth, I.A.P. (1988) *Containing Anxiety in Institutions*. Free Association Books, London.

NHSE (2000) *Nursing in Prison*. DoH, London.

Orwell, G. (1989) *Nineteen Eighty Four*. Penguin, London.

Page, S. and Woskett, V. (1994) *Supervising the Counsellor*. Routledge, London.

Parker, I. (1999) (ed.) *Deconstructing Psychotherapy*. Sage, London.

Proctor, B. (1986) Supervision: a co-operative exercise in accountability. In *Enabling and Ensuring* (Marken, M. & Payne, M., eds), pp. 118–27. National Youth Bureau and Council for Education and Training in Youth and Community Work, Leicester.

Rolfe, G., Freshwater, D. and Jasper, M. (2001) *Critical Reflection for Nurses and the Caring Professions: A User's Guide*. Palgrave, Basingstoke.

Swain, G. (1995) *Clinical Supervision: The Principles and Process*. Community Practitioners and Health Visitors Association, London.

UKCC (1992) *Code of Professional Conduct*. UKCC, London.

UKCC (1996) *Position Statement on Clinical Supervision*. UKCC, London.

Virilio, P. (1996) *Cybermonde: La Politique du Pire*. Textuel, Paris.

Winnicott, D.W. (1991) *The Maturational Processes and the Facilitating Environment*. Hogarth, London.

Chapter 6

Developing Prison Health Care through Reflective Practice

Liz Walsh

Introduction

The aim of this chapter is to examine the potential for practice development in prison health care through the use of reflective practice and the implementation of clinical supervision. In order for the reader to be able to put the discussion into context, it is necessary to have an understanding of the particular nature of nursing in a prison. It is also important to be aware of the recent and ongoing changes in prison health care, at both national and local level. This is because the nature and context of prison nursing, when viewed in the light of the major policy changes that have been and are being implemented, have an impact on service delivery and staff motivation. In the current climate of change and evolution in prison health care, the effective use of reflection would be highly beneficial. What follows is an examination of the prison context and the role of the nurse in prison health care, and a discussion of policy and service changes and their impact on prison nurses. The benefits of reflective practice in this setting will be discussed, as will a study I was involved with as part of a research team concerned with the introduction of clinical supervision into this environment. Finally, I will draw on my own previous experiences as a nurse working in prison and my role as a practice developer in prison health care in examining the issues involved in promoting and using reflective practice to develop nursing practice in prisons.

The context of prison nursing

Not all nurses have an interest in prison health care. However, most nurses at some time have cared or will care for a prisoner or a member of that person's family.

At the time of writing there are just over 73 000 people in prison in England and Wales, male and female, ranging from the age of 15 upwards (HM Prison Service 2003). It is estimated that over 1 million people per year are affected by imprisonment, either as prisoners themselves or as someone with a family member in prison. The health care needs of this population are similar to those in the community. However, it has been suggested that 90% of the prison population have a diagnosable mental health problem (including personality disorder) or substance misuse problem or both, and 80% of prisoners smoke (NHS Executive & HM Prison Service 2001). In addition to the possible pre-existing health needs of prisoner-patients there are health needs created as a consequence of imprisonment. Examples of these include the lack of direct access to over-the-counter medications, restriction on family networks/support, overcrowding and limited opportunities for self-care.

Health care in prison is provided by a multidisciplinary team comprising doctors, nurses, health care officers, physiotherapists, chiropodists, dentists, radiographers, specialist nurses, opticians, etc. Interestingly, the multidisciplinary team in a prison comprises a far wider spectrum of professionals than in the outside world. For example, the nurse/health care officer in the prison setting may also liaise with probation officers, discipline (prison) officers, chaplains, psychologists, physical education staff and other educational staff in caring for a prisoner.

Registered nurses and health care officers provide nursing care in prison. Health care officers can be viewed as 'specialist' prison officers. These specialist prison officers have undertaken a 6-month training course provided by the prison service in basic health care and nursing. Some of these prison officers may also be registered nurses but some are not. Since 2003, the traditional Prison Service health care officer training has been replaced by an NVQ level 3 in Custodial Health Care delivered in conjunction with external educational providers.

Registered nurses working in prison who are not trained as health care officers are relatively new to the Prison Service. It is only since the 1980s that nurses without health care officer or indeed prison officer training have been employed by the Service. There are currently over 1000 nurses working in prisons in England and Wales.

The role of the nurse in a prison is varied and complex. Prisoners present a range of health problems, often spanning the spectrum of traditional nursing specialities. Hence, nurses working in prison need skills in mental health nursing, general nursing (both medical and surgical), primary care/practice nursing, learning disability nursing and children's nursing (for those nurses working with young offenders). This presents a professional challenge to practitioners, educationalists and researchers alike. Not only are nurses working in prison providing nursing care to the prison population but they also have a role similar to that of the prison officer in maintaining security and order. This demands skills and competencies in both nursing care and security.

The prison population can be viewed as a small community representative of the community outside prison. Prison staff can therefore expect to deal with chronic illness, mental illness, drug and alcohol misuse, acute medical problems and trauma. In addition, nursing staff also provide health screening services for all prisoners entering the prison system, and inpatient services for both medical, surgical and psychiatric care. In addition to this, nurses and health care officers also provide well man clinics, chronic disease management clinics and primary health care/practice nursing similar to that provided at a local GP surgery.

Care and custody

It is widely recognised that nursing in a prison presents the nurse with a wide range of challenges and frustrations that affect nursing practice. Much of this results from the dual caring and security role that the nurse undertakes in this setting (Freshwater *et al.* 2002a). In addition to the dual role of carer and custodian, the nurse also has to practise within the culture of the prison setting. It is important to remember that the main function of a prison is security/rehabilitation and not health care.

Anecdotal literature suggests that the dual role of the nurse and the prison environment pose unique problems and challenges to the nurse. Much of the published work concerning nurses working in the prison environment is anecdotal (see Box 6.1). Although empirical literature is limited, it supports much of what is discussed in the anecdotal reports.

A scoping study commissioned by the UKCC (UKCC & University of Central Lancashire 1999) was the first major research study to examine nursing in a secure environment. This aimed to examine:

- The competencies required of nurses working in secure environments.
- The extent to which nursing interventions in secure environments are evidence based.
- The current activity in the development of practice standards in secure environments with specific reference to particular client groups.
- The preparation given to nurses working in secure environments.
- The issues faced by nurses working in secure environments which may compromise therapeutic relationships with particular reference to personality disordered patients.
- The extent to which current Council policies are utilised and inform practice.
- Practice issues relevant to the physical health needs of specific populations within secure environments, e.g. care of women, or of people from different cultural backgrounds.

This study gathered evidence that demonstrated a low level of clinical supervision, which was attributed in part to practical problems and a lack of management support. The authors highlighted the sense of isolation felt by practitioners as a result of the lack of clinical supervision, and also reported a lack of formal and informal mentorship/preceptorship arrangements.

Another British study commissioned by the RCN Prison Nurses Forum (Dale & Woods 2001) aimed to provide a comprehensive overview of the roles and boundaries of practice of nurses working in prison. Following an extensive literature review, the study utilised observational case studies, focus groups and consensus conferences for data collection. In addition to these data collection methods, re-analysis of the data presented in the report by the UKCC & the University of Central Lancashire (1999) was also undertaken. This project highlighted the competencies required by nurses working in prisons whilst noting the different types of health care centres in which these nurses

Box 6.1   Published works concerning nurses in the prison environment

Alexander-Rodriguez, T. (1983) Prison health: A role for professional nursing. *Nursing Outlook*, **31**(2): 115–18.

Day, R.A. (1983) The challenge: health care vs security. *The Canadian Nurse*, **79**(7): 34–6.

Holleran, C. (1983) Ethics in prison health care. *International Nursing Review*, **30**(5): 138–45.

Dopson, L. (1988) Beds behind bars. *Nursing Times*, **84**(19): 35–7.

Reeder, D. (1991) Conceptualising psychosocial nursing in the jail setting. *Journal of Psychosocial Nursing*, **29**(8): 40–3.

Dulfer, S. (1992) No holds barred. *Nursing*, **5**(4): 20–2.

Mason, P. & Adam, S. (1992) Breaking into prisons. *Health Service Journal*, 16 January: 22.

Burrow, S. (1993) The role conflict of the forensic nurse. *Senior Nurse*, **13**(5): 20–5.

Stevens, R. (1993) When your clients are in jail. *Nursing Forum*, **28**(4): 4–5.

Willmott, Y. (1994) Career opportunities in the nursing service for prisoners. *Nursing Times*, **90**(24): 29–30.

Barr, J. (1995) Pressure on prison nurses from non-qualified staff. *Nursing Standard*, **9**(45): 17.

Burrows, R. (1995) Captive care: changes in prison nursing. *Nursing Standard*, **9**(22): 29–31.

Peternelj-Taylor, C. & Johnson, R. (1995) Serving time: psychiatric mental health nursing in corrections. *Journal of Psychosocial Nursing*, **33**(8): 12–19.

Rodgers, P. & Topping-Morris, B. (1996) Prison and the role of the forensic mental health nurse. *Nursing Times*, **92**(31): 32–5.

Wilmott, Y. (1996) Duty bound. *Nursing Standard*, **10**(13): 6.

Lyne, M. (1997) No bars on nursing care. *Nursing Standard*, **12**(11): 18.

McMillan, I. (1997) Behind bars. *Nursing Times*, **93**(10): 14–15.

Schafer, P. (1997) When a client develops an attraction: successful resolution versus boundary violation. *Journal of Psychiatric and Mental Health Nursing*, **4**: 203–11.

Willmott, Y. (1997) Prison nursing: the tension between custody and care. *British Journal of Nursing*, **6**(6): 333–6.

Reams, P., Neff Smith, M., Fletcher, J. & Spencer, E. (1988) Making the case for bioethics in corrections. *Corrections Today*, April: 112–17, 176.

Norman, A. & Parrish, A. (1999a) Prison nursing. *Nursing Management*, **6**(6): 8–9.

Norman, A. & Parrish, A. (1999b) Prison health care: work environment and the nursing role. *British Journal of Nursing*, **8**(10): 653–9.

Smith, C. (2000) 'Healthy prisons': a contradiction in terms? *The Howard Journal*, **39**(4): 339–53.

Parrish, A. (2002) Prison health care: who needs a nurse? *Nursing Management*, **8**(8): 6–9.

work. The difficulties experienced by prison nurses were also emphasised, and were reported to be centred around the nature of the environment where the primary purpose is security, not health care. Indeed, security often takes precedence over all other considerations including, at times, health care. Nurses included in this study also reported the nursing role in prisons as being more about breadth than depth as nurses in prison are providing care from many specialities including mental health, general nursing, occupational health and primary care. The nurses questioned felt that the unique culture of the prison environment is not well suited to the traditional values of professional nursing practice.

Gulotta (1986) examined the factors influencing nursing practice and job satisfaction in prison hospitals in America, where they are referred to as correctional hospitals. Fifty registered nurses who had worked in the correctional setting for at least six months were studied using a survey methodology in which two questionnaires were administered. This study found that, for the correctional health care setting studied, the nursing administration, hospital administration, nursing practice ability and nursing role, as defined on the questionnaire, facilitated nursing practice. It was also discovered that the correctional administration was the least facilitating factor to nursing practice and had fewer correlations with job satisfaction than with any other variable. Nurses in this study felt that the goals of the correctional administration and the nursing service were in opposition. This implies that the goals of security and nursing are in conflict with one another, leading to a care versus custody dilemma that is highlighted frequently in the anecdotal literature.

In the study by Gulotta (1986) high levels of job satisfaction were found in this group of nurses. These were attributed to the uniqueness of the setting. Gulotta recommended that there should be a balance between security constraints and inmates' health care needs. This, the author concluded, could be facilitated through good communication and co-operation between health care and correctional staff. Gulotta (1986) also recommended a programme of health awareness for correctional staff to provide an insight into the operation of health care services within a correctional setting.

Droes (1994) explored the nature and problems of nursing practice in a correctional setting in America. She employed a qualitative method involving participant observation, of which there was in excess of 100 hours, together with informal interviews and conversations. Three men's prisons were studied, and Droes interviewed 40 nursing staff. Two broad questions guided the study, namely what is the nature and what are the problems of nursing practice in a correctional setting. Two different groups of nursing staff participated in this study. Forty registered nurses employed in three prisons participated in informal interviews and conversations. Also included in this study were five nurses who had current or past experience in seven additional prison and jail settings who were personally known to the researcher. They were interviewed formally and at length outside the correctional setting. Droes discovered three important facets of nursing in a correctional setting: first, the special world in which nursing work occurs; second, the actual correctional nursing work; and finally the correctional health care scenes – the interactions that occur among various individuals and groups and influence correctional nursing practice.

In discussing what she refers to as 'the special world' in which the nursing work occurs, Droes (1994) explained that the structural conditions of the correctional setting hold consequences for nursing care to inmates. Structural conditions are elaborated further in three areas:

(1) the ever-present security measures
(2) inadequate facilities, equipment and supplies
(3) insufficient staffing.

Droes highlighted the ever-present security measures as the most profoundly influencing factor in the delivery of nursing care.

Droes found that the interactions between various individuals and groups within the correctional setting hold consequences for nursing practice. She discovered that custody's toleration of health care was most notable in the interactions between custody staff and health care staff. Droes described a continuum of toleration of health care staff by custody staff. At one end of the continuum, contentious toleration of health care occurred where 'custody staff accepted inmate health care grudgingly and viewed it as a distraction and interference with the performance of their own work' (Droes 1994, p. 204). At the other end of this continuum, according to Droes, there was toleration which 'denoted situations in which custody staff evaluated health care as not only benefiting inmates but also assisting in the performance of their own work' (p. 205). Droes mentions an acknowledged toleration at the centre of this continuum in which custody staff 'perceived correctional health care as meeting reasonable needs and as a routinised and accepted aspect of correctional work' (p. 204).

From the data Droes (1994) concluded that the nurses had differing conceptions of nursing although they fell into three broad categories. Some nurses had a limited conception of nursing in which they tended to focus on acute medical and surgical problems. Others held an expanded conception in which they included the narrow, acute medical/surgical nursing but also included a public health and social–psychological approach to health care problems. Droes also mentioned a third group of nurses holding a different conception of nursing, namely 'other directed' nurses. She stated that they 'held conceptions of nursing that tended to reflect the prevailing views of influentials within the correctional health care scene' (p. 205).

Droes drew two main conclusions: first, that custody staff exert significant influence on the correctional health care environment; and, second, that nurses working in the correctional environment with increased levels of education and experience in public health are prepared to provide a broader scope of health care to inmates. Therefore, the most favourable conditions for health care delivery in prisons occurred when there was a considered toleration by correctional officers and an expanded conception of nursing by nurses.

Droes (1994) noted that caution must be applied in generalising these results to other correctional settings because of the characteristics of the sites and the respondents. However, there are underlying themes in this study that are consistent with both empirical and anecdotal literature, both nationally and internationally.

In an Australian study, Doyle (1999) examined the factors influencing the practice of psychiatric nursing in an Australian prison. A qualitative methodology was adopted for this study in which 10 psychiatric nurses working in the prison setting were asked in a focus group to identify and explore issues of concern in their practice in the prison setting. Following the focus group, themes identified were explored further by the use of in-depth interviewing, using open-ended questions and non-directive language techniques. Twenty nurses were interviewed, the initial ten from the focus group plus another ten who had expressed an interest in the study. Interviews were tape-recorded, transcribed and analysed using thematic textual analysis. Clusters of themes were identified and the emergent understandings were returned to the subjects for clarification and comment.

Doyle (1999) reported the following factors as influencing psychiatric nursing in the prison setting: challenging patients, threats to the personal survival of patients, the technology and artifice of confinement, conflicting values of correctional and nursing staff, stigma by association and prisoner identification of the nurses within the prison administration. He concluded that psychiatric nurses working in the Australian prison system are practising in an environment where the philosophy and values of correction and criminal justice intrude on nursing practice goals and their outcomes. Doyle recommended ongoing further research in this setting to inform changes in prison-based practice. The findings from this study confirm what is highlighted in the anecdotal literature. That is, the intrusion of a correctional/prison philosophy into core nursing values causes professional difficulties for the prison/correctional nurse.

It is widely recognised in both the empirical and anecdotal literature that nursing in a prison presents the nurse with a wide range of challenges and frustrations that affect nursing practice in prison. Much of this is thought to result from the dual caring and security role that the nurse undertakes in this setting. In addition to the dual role of carer and custodian, the nurse also has to practise within the culture of the prison setting. It is important to remember that the main function of a prison is security/rehabilitation and not health care (Horner & Stacey 1999 cited in Willcox 2002; Norman & Parrish 2002). What follows are a few examples of the issues that having a dual role raises for the prison nurse.

The nurse–patient relationship in a prison setting is one in which it is felt that boundaries are vital. As Norman and Parrish (2002, p. 15) state, 'Many of the clients with whom prison nurses work may present specific challenges with regard to manipulative behaviours that can be designed to compromise and undermine the essence of nursing care.' This is supported by Schafer (1997, p. 205) in her paper concerning boundary violations in the correctional setting. She states that:

> Correctional nurses encounter an environment where their clients employ manipulative and intimidating behaviours, and personal safety may be threatened. Hence, the correctional culture, coupled with a history of oppression, creates an atmosphere ripe for the potential to exploit and be exploited.

Chapman (1980) suggests that both the nurse and the patient have rights and responsibilities within the nurse–patient relationship. The nurse has the right to co-operation, gratitude, recognition and a happy environment. The patient has a right to receive skilled nursing care, individual recognition and information. The responsibilities of the nurse are to provide skilled, individualised, non-judgemental care, to promote health, to alleviate suffering, to prevent illness and to restore health. The patient too has responsibilities: to co-operate, to recognise the nurse as an individual and to be grateful and open in communication. It is suggested that being open in communication refers to the concept of trust within the nurse–patient relationship. If each of the rights and responsibilities is examined within the context of the prisoner/patient–nurse relationship, it can be demonstrated that, because of the security element of the prison nurse's job and the nature of the environment, not all rights and responsibilities can be met by both parties. For example, if a prisoner/patient prefers to be located in the hospital wing of the prison, it will sometimes be in the patient's interest not to co-operate with health care advice given by the nurse if taking the advice means the prisoner/patient will recover and be moved from the health care centre to the main prison. Another example concerns the trust that should be inherent in a nurse–patient relationship. If a prisoner/patient wants to misuse painkillers, he/she will have to pretend to be in pain to elicit the painkillers from the doctor and then from the nurse. It will be the nurse and doctor who will have to decide if the patient is telling the truth about the extent and severity of their pain. This can be difficult in the prison setting. In unpublished material (Walsh 1998) it was noted that mistrust of prisoner/patients is common in prison health care, and that nurses find they have to rely heavily on their experience and intuition when dealing with them. Burrow (1993, p. 23) states that this is a common problem in nursing in secure environments, and comments:

> the forensic nurse must exercise a benign scepticism. This is not to say that a patient's wishes are not to be entertained but that an awareness should exist that they may be actively exploited to undermine the integrity of security procedures and gain some personal advantage.

It is not suggested that this issue is unique to prison nurses as there are many nurses working in other secure environments where they have an important contribution to make in terms of security. However, prison is the only secure environment in which nurses work where health is not the primary focus. Special hospitals such as Broadmoor (UK) and regional secure units also have security as an important part of the nurse's role. However, secure health provision is the main focus as all their clients are patients whereas the prison nurse deals with all aspects of a prisoner's health, not just when he/she is an inpatient.

It has been well documented that the culture within which prison nurses work has a great impact on their practice (Schafer 1997; Norman & Parrish 2002; Willcox 2002). Stevens (1993) in an anecdotal article highlights the collision of cultures that nurses can experience when nursing in a secure environment. Table 6.1, from Stevens (1993), illustrates the two main cultures prevalent in a prison in which health care is not the primary focus.

Table 6.1   Two main cultures prevalent in a prison where health care is not the primary focus

Element	Health care	Prison
Values	Basic goodness All individuals are essentially the same	Evil is present Criminal traits exist
Beliefs	Individuals who say they are sick should receive attention People obey the rules	Individuals who say they are sick are trying to get out of something People break the rules
Norms	Respect the patient Get the patients well and home	Distrust the inmate Get the individuals convicted and incarcerated
	Anger and hostility are acceptable behaviours when a person is ill. Assistance is offered, anger is redirected Resisting treatment calls for counselling with restraints being the last resort	Anger and hostility are not acceptable. Hostile inmates necessitate higher security Resisting arrest is not tolerated and restraints are the first resort (handcuffs)
	Assumption of danger to self is minimal	Assumption of danger to self is ever present

Current policy development

There have been major changes in prison health care in the past decade. The most radical of changes began with a publication by Her Majesty's Chief Inspector of Prisons, Sir David Ramsbotham. Ramsbotham published a discussion paper following the publication of inspection reports that, in terms of health care, highlighted 'a number of major deficiencies and problems in actual delivery that need to be addressed' (HMIP 1996, Foreword). The discussion paper has as its terms of reference 'to consider health care arrangements in Prison Service establishments in England and Wales with a view to ensuring that prisoners are given the same access to the same quality and range of health care services as the general public receives from the National Health Service' (HMIP 1996, Terms of Reference). The report examined the concept of the prisoner as a patient. It asked if the prisoner with health care needs was seen as a prisoner or as a patient and how their health care needs might best be met. In this discussion paper, the Chief Inspector of Prisons recommended that 'it is no longer sensible to maintain a health care service for prisoners separate from the NHS' (HMIP 1996, p. 7). The discussion paper also stated that 'there is an immediate need for the Home Office and the Department of Health, together with the Prison Service and the National Health Service, to agree a timetable for the NHS to assume responsibility for the commissioning and provision of health care and health promotion in prisons' (HMIP 1996, p. 7).

   Traditionally, prison health care was provided by the prison service through the Directorate of Health Care at the Prison Service. HM Prison

Service itself is part of the Home Office. Following publication of this discussion paper a working party was established with representation from both the NHS Executive and HM Prison Service to examine the recommendations. The report of this working party was published in 1999 (NHS Executive & HM Prison Service 1999) and endorsed the aim of providing access to the same range and quality of health care for prisoners as is available in the NHS. However, at that time the report did not support the recommendation that responsibility for commissioning and provision of health care belong to the NHS. Moreover, the working party recommended that 'health care in prisons [be] delivered through a formal partnership between the NHS and the Prison Service' (HMIP 1996, p. 17). As a consequence, a formal partnership was established between the Prison Service and the NHS, and the Prison Health Policy Unit and Task Force were created. The Prison Health Policy Unit replaced the old Directorate of Health Care and assumed responsibility to develop prison health policy which would integrate and draw on existing NHS policy. The Task Force was established to support prisons and health authorities in the development of services, assessment of prisoner health care needs and the changes identified in the prison health improvement programmes.

The working party report also considered the future organisation of prison health care and ways in which to improve provision. As part of this, health care staffing was examined, as was the culture within which health care was being provided. In addressing issues of culture, the report mentioned that the health care culture was influenced by traditional attitudes with an emphasis on security and less on nursing practice and health improvement. In this context, the report states that

> newly recruited nurses often found it difficult to influence the culture that lacked clear lines of accountability to support them. These factors reduced job satisfaction and contributed to poor retention of nursing staff.

> (NHS Executive & HM Prison Service 1999, p. 11)

During the same period the large-scale research study commissioned by the United Kingdom Central Council for Nursing and Midwifery (UKCC & University of Central Lancashire 1999) was set up to scope the issues involved in the work of practitioners working in secure environments. This study made many recommendations and reached conclusions concerning nursing in prison health care. One of the most significant was similar to that from the working party in that it was noted that health care culture is influenced by traditional attitudes emphasising security before nursing practice and health improvement. The report found this particularly evident where senior members of staff had been in post for several years and were not qualified nurses.

This report also mentioned the lack of clinical supervision opportunities for nursing staff working in prison health care. It mentioned that there was a low level of provision of clinical supervision, and it was felt that this was possibly due to practical problems and a lack of management support creating implementation difficulties.

Following the publication of *Nursing in Secure Environments* (UKCC & University of Central Lancashire 1999), and public concern regarding health care in prison, the Prisons Minister and the Health Minister set up a working party to look at the development of nursing in prisons in England and Wales with specific reference to health care officers. The report published by the working party (NHS Executive & HM Prison Service 2000) provided recommendations for the training and induction of health care officers and new nurses and also the development of health care managers in prisons. It was as a result of this report that health care officer training was revised and replaced by the NVQ in Custodial Health Care.

It can be seen that there have been major changes in prison health since the publication of *Patient or Prisoner* (HMIP 1996). This discussion document instigated a major restructuring of prison health care at a national level in the development of a partnership model. Since the setting up of the partnership, it has developed further with more services being delivered by the NHS inside prisons in England and Wales, e.g. the introduction of NHS mental health in-reach teams which were developed as part of the NHS Plan (NHS Executive 2000).

In September 2002 a statement was issued by the Home Secretary and the Secretary of State for Health stating that from April 2003 funding responsibility for prison health services would be transferred from the Home Office to the Department of Health. This is the first step in a five-year plan whereby NHS Primary Care Trusts will become responsible for the commissioning and provision of health-care services to prisoners in their areas. The transfer of prison health to the NHS brings with it exciting developments for nursing staff currently working within prisons. It is expected that there will be more scope for the professional development of both prison health care staff and staff in the wider NHS as a result of these changes.

Reflective practice in prison health care

Upon taking up the post of prison nurse lecturer practitioner, it became clear to me that although the concept of reflective practice and clinical supervision had been high on the nursing agenda for many years, it was relatively rare in prison health care. Indeed, this was one of the findings from the Nursing in Secure Environments project (UKCC & University of Central Lancashire 1999). The report mentioned that there was a low level of acceptance of clinical supervision in the prison setting and that it was not readily available to nurses in prison working in conditions that tested their professional resilience. This report also mentioned that 'the patient groups and professional isolation, in some instances, would suggest that this is an area where nurses would benefit from the rigorous and systematic application of clinical supervision' (UKCC & University of Central Lancashire 1999, p. 105).

As a result of the findings of the UKCC & University of Central Lancashire (1999) and concern regarding the lack of clinical supervision in the prisons in my area, a project team examining the implementation of clinical supervision in prison health care in another area of the country was contacted. A project, which would encompass the cluster of prisons with which I was working, was then established. I do not intend to provide the reader with an in-depth report of this research project as that can be found in other literature (Freshwater *et al.* 2002a; 2002b).

In total, five prisons were invited to participate in the project. Each prison was asked to identify staff who would be interested in becoming clinical supervisors. These staff were then given training in clinical supervision with a view to becoming supervisors. The training was undertaken by the project team; however, the fifth prison used an external consultant to prepare the supervisors. The preparation given to four of the prisons comprised three days' training over one month. The external consultant used by the fifth prison was contacted to ascertain the content of the training to ensure its consistency throughout the prisons. Demographic data was collected from the sample of supervisors involved in the initial training. The newly trained supervisors in two of the prisons were given access to an external supervisor who facilitated group supervision on a regular basis following the period of initial training. This support was provided to augment the initial training given and to increase the confidence of the newly trained supervisors.

Clinical supervision was then implemented in the participating prisons and evaluated using semistructured tape-recorded interviews, telephone interviews and the use of the Manchester Clinical Supervision Scale (see Freshwater *et al.* 2002b).

The total number of staff involved in the project was 35 in five prisons, as follows: 2 external supervisors, 16 supervisors in the five prisons, 4 health-care managers and 13 supervisees.

Three themes emerged from the evaluation of the implementation of clinical supervision in these prisons, namely practice, education and barriers to implementation.

Practice

Staff mentioned the following four issues concerning the practice of clinical supervision in their prisons: timing of clinical supervision, time for clinical supervision, location of sessions and trust/safety/confidentiality.

Timing of clinical supervision

There were marked differences in the frequency and duration of clinical supervision sessions expected by staff in the prisons. Twenty minutes once a month was felt to be appropriate in one prison whilst other establishments were looking to have one hour per week.

Time for clinical supervision

It was felt that there was not enough time during the working day for staff to participate in or to provide clinical supervision sessions. Some managers offered staff time off in lieu for attending sessions, some agreed to pay over-time, whilst others suggested that, if supervisor and supervisee ensured that they worked the same shifts, time could be made available. Prisons operate a rigid shift pattern and this was mentioned as being a problem.

Location of sessions

The preferred location of supervision sessions varied amongst prisons. Some staff suggested they would prefer to have supervision sessions away from the prison as it would mean fewer distractions and they would find it easier to talk. Other staff said they felt it to be more beneficial to have the sessions inside the prison so they would be available in the event of an emergency, and they felt it would be simpler than leaving the prison.

Trust/safety/confidentiality

Some staff reported that they did not feel comfortable discussing their practice in the prison setting. Issues such as the culture of blame that was perceived to exist in some prisons was mentioned as it led some staff to feel unsafe. Some staff also felt that their supervision sessions might not be confidential, and there was mention of a feeling of 'Big Brother watching' in some instances.

Education

It was mentioned by some staff that the prison setting is not an environment in which learning and education are part of the culture unless it is mandatory training that is provided by the prison itself. Confidence and confusion were the two main themes which were highlighted.

Confidence

In terms of the preparation given to supervisors prior to their taking up the role of supervisor, it was felt that the training provided gave some staff the confidence to run one-to-one supervision sessions but not group sessions. Interestingly, some supervisees felt that attending clinical supervision sessions actually gave them more confidence in practice and helped reduce feelings of isolation.

Confusion

There was confusion amongst the supervisees concerning the purpose of clinical supervision and the role of mentors, preceptors and post-incident debriefing in the clinical setting.

Barriers

There were three main themes that emerged when looking at the evaluation data concerning the implementation of clinical supervision sessions. These comprised operational issues, personnel issues and cultural/institutional issues.

Operational issues

In discussions concerning the lack of time available for staff to participate in sessions some participants felt that the rigid regime present in the prison setting is a barrier to facilitating clinical supervision. Low staffing levels in some of the establishments also made it difficult to undertake clinical supervision as staff could not take time out. A heavy workload was stated as another reason why staff could not take time to have clinical supervision.

Personnel issues

It was felt that in some of the prisons there was very poor communication between staff and management, and that this hampered attempts to implement clinical supervision in terms of arranging time and understanding the pressures staff faced when trying to facilitate supervision sessions. Apathy and lack of motivation were also cited by some participants as the reason for lack of supervision in their establishments. A culture of blame and suspicion appeared to be present in some establishments which, when added to apathy and lack of motivation, caused barriers to successful implementation.

Cultural/institutional issues

From the evidence gained during evaluation of the implementation of clinical supervision in this setting, it appeared that there was a cultural/institutional element to the lack of implementation in some of the prisons. It was felt that there was sabotage by some staff against those staff who were working hard to implement sessions. There appeared to be cynicism about clinical supervision and its benefits in this setting, born out of suspicion (see Chapter 5).

Summary

This study raises some interesting insights into the culture of the prison health care setting at the time. It not only highlights the need for a culture of reflection in the prison setting, but also demonstrates the problems of promoting and facilitating such an environment. Reflective practice as a part of clinical supervision is evident. However, implementing clinical supervision into some of the prison settings in the study proved to be fraught with difficulty. Taking a step back from implementing clinical supervision and promoting an environment of reflection has also proved difficult in some prisons. Informal anecdotal evidence suggests that the traditional culture of the prison setting does not readily lend itself to the philosophy of reflection. This is not to say that all prison health care staff are averse to undertaking reflection in and on action. Far from it. However, this culture is more evident and stronger in some establishments than in others, and the culture within the health care staff is influenced to a large extent by the quality of the leadership present. In some settings in which managers are relatively new to the prison service or naturally have the ability to challenge 'custom and practice' and manage change effectively, reflective practice is beginning to emerge. In some establishments clinical supervision is flourishing, and the effects on staff morale and patient care can be witnessed clearly.

The clinical supervision study referred to in this chapter was undertaken at a time when prison health care was beginning to change significantly. However, staff were unsure as to the future of health care in prisons and were working at a time when national changes were beginning to filter into local policy. The issues raised can therefore be understood quite clearly when viewed in this context.

The following reflection of my own, broadly using Johns' model of structured reflection (Johns 1998), illustrates some of the issues that may underlie the reluctance of some staff to accept clinical supervision comfortably. It also demonstrates the potential for reflective practice in prison health care.

A personal reflection

"I was on night duty when I was called to one of the residential wings to see a prisoner who was complaining of feeling unwell. I was escorted from the health care centre to the wing by a senior prison officer, as is usual practice on night duty, where we met with a prison officer on the wing where the prisoner was located. I knew the prisoner from an admission he had had to the medical inpatient unit of the prison the previous week. I remembered that he had not wanted to be moved back to the residential wing from the health care centre when he was declared fit for discharge by the doctor. He had told us he still felt unwell but his tests showed his illness had resolved and he was no longer unwell enough to be in the health care centre as an inpatient. I had built up a fairly good professional relationship with this prisoner whilst he was an inpatient and felt as though there was a degree of trust between us. We had had a busy night in the prison and the senior prison officer also was clearly busy. As I knew the recent medical history of this prisoner I took some medication I thought might be useful in case he could be treated in his cell. I also took some equipment with me so that I could perform some observations on him if necessary. As we approached the wing I told the officer who accompanied me that I already knew the prisoner as I had worked with him before. The three of us approached the prisoner's cell with the senior officer first so he could unlock the door. When the prisoner saw me he looked somewhat relieved and proceeded to tell me the problem. Using my prior experience and knowledge of the prisoner, I decided that he should come back to the inpatient unit so that I could observe him more closely overnight and so that he could see the doctor first thing in the morning on his round. I felt that although to relocate the prisoner to the inpatient unit in the middle of the night would be awkward in terms of security, it would be better for all concerned in the long run. I would be able to undertake some further tests that I felt were necessary to eliminate some concerns I had, and I would be able to observe him more closely than if he was left on the wing. I knew that if he was left on the wing he would ring his call bell constantly as he was in some discomfort, and that the officers would have to keep escorting me to the wing to open his cell. In my clinical opinion, this prisoner needed more care than could be provided on the wing. Once I had finished assessing the prisoner, I stepped outside the cell where the officers were standing, to explain to them why I wanted him moved into the health care centre for the rest of the night.

My request was greeted with some annoyance and irritation. I was told that in their opinion this prisoner was lying and he was fine. They felt he just wanted to be moved back into the health care centre, possibly because he was in debt on the wing. Although I could understand why they thought the way they did, and I too had a few reservations, I felt that they were not in possession of the knowledge I had of the prisoner as my patient the previous week. The officers did not want him moved as they did not think he was unwell and because of the security risk. I spent a few minutes talking to the officers, explaining my concerns. My clinical judgement was continually questioned. I was at least 20 years younger than the senior officer and I was a female nurse who had only been qualified for a couple of years. Here I was, faced with two male prison officers with a great deal of experience in prison, disagreeing with them. This discussion was only terminated when I had explained the concept of my professional accountability to them and mentioned my strong desire not to be called to a coroner's court should anything happen to the prisoner. The prisoner was moved into the health care inpatient unit against the wishes of the officers.

I handed over to the day staff the following morning and explained what had happened. I explained that the officers had expressed reservations about the authenticity of the prisoner/patient's complaint but that I was not willing to take any risks in the night as he had been unwell previously. When I returned that evening for my shift, the prisoner was gone: back to the wing. 'Nothing wrong with him,' they told me."

Aesthetics

Throughout this whole incident I was trying to achieve the best possible care for the prisoner whilst maintaining a good relationship with my prison officer colleagues. I responded as I did for these reasons. The consequences of my actions for those involved were as follows. For the patient, he was moved to the health care centre and was provided with the care and observation that I believed he needed. For the other people involved, i.e. the prison officers, the move from the wing to the health care centre provided more work as moving a prisoner during the night has security implications that need to be taken into consideration and can make the process more time consuming. For myself, the consequences were many-fold. First, I had an extra patient to care for overnight. However, perhaps the most important consequence for me personally was the reputation I gained with my discipline colleagues. Also important to me was the perception the prisoner now had of me. I felt I was now seen by both my prison officer colleagues and the prisoner to be on the latter's side. I was treading a fine line with my officer colleagues as I had overruled their opinion and insisted that my professional opinion be accepted. It appeared to me that the prisoner felt I would do whatever he asked of me. Once we had moved into the health care centre and the officers had left, I had to discuss my actions with him and made it very clear as to my reasons for moving him. Boundaries were set and reinforced regarding his behaviour and my plan for his treatment. It seemed that the prisoner was relieved that he was now in the health care centre, and felt that there was opportunity for personal gain for him. Consequently he seemed quite happy and did not appear to be as unwell as when I first saw him on the wing.

Personal issues

Initially I felt as though I was in control of the situation. However, once I had made the decision to move the prisoner, my feelings changed slightly as a result of the response I received from the prison officers. Instead of being left to get on with my job with the support of my colleagues, I now had to argue with my officer colleagues and defend my clinical decision. I felt that I had to remain calm and professional, but I did become angry inside as I felt intimidated by them. I also knew that, if the officers refused to work with me and would not move the prisoner, then there would be very little I could do for my patient. Here, I felt, were major issues of power, authority and organisational culture. It was a perfect example of the care/custody philosophy clash in action. Once the officers had agreed to move the prisoner, not only was I concerned that my working relationship with them for that night would be difficult but also that we still had more nights to work together. The outcome of the prisoner's consultation with the doctor the next morning would be known to all the night staff the following night and I knew that these officers would be very interested to know if they had been right or not. The prisoner's location the following night would speak volumes and have a huge impact on my clinical reputation. This was a stressful thought.

Ethics

I feel that my actions matched with my beliefs about how patients should be treated and cared for in this environment. I also feel that my beliefs about the importance of working in the best interests of the patient were evident in my actions. During my decision making, it did cross my mind that the prisoner might be lying to me and might just have wanted to move back to health care. However, after weighing up the consequences of the possible outcomes I decided that I could not risk leaving the prisoner on the wing without treatment. I was prepared for the consequences of my actions had I been wrong and the officers been right. I decided that my professional integrity and accountability must come first.

Empirics

My nurse training and previous work informed my professional knowledge in this situation with this patient. I knew and understood his illness from his previous admission and had been closely involved in his care. My knowledge of my professional code of practice also had a major impact on the decisions I made that night.

Reflexivity

The experience of that night was not new to me. I had learnt from previous experiences and from having witnessed what happened to other nurse colleagues that erring on the side of caution and going against the wishes and opinions of officer colleagues when making decisions about patients can cause the nurse's reputation to be tarnished. However, I also knew that, in the eyes of some officers, civilian nurses in prison would always be seen as 'soft touch'. Thus I knew that with some officers, whatever I did, this group reputation would not change. I also felt that it really did not matter to me what they thought of me as I had a job to do and the patient was my priority. This is not to say that I did not listen to the officers. I believe that we should work as a multidisciplinary team and as such the opinions of all team members are equally valid. However, in this situation I felt that the responsibility for the patient was mine, and that should anything untoward have happened to him I would be accountable. Having reflected on this incident numerous times, I still feel as though I did the right thing at the time and would do the same again.

If I had not acted as I did and left the prisoner in his cell, I feel that the officers would have been much happier. Knowing what I know now, I suspect that, had I left the prisoner on the wing, he would have continued to ring his cell bell throughout the night as he knew I was on duty and would be called to see him. Personally, if I had left this prisoner in his cell after having already been called to see him and expressed concern, I would have spent the night and the next day worrying that I had made the wrong decision and I would have been concerned for his well being.

When I think about this experience now, I feel angry that I was put in the position in the first place. In my role as practice developer I also feel concerned for some of the nurses who are still in the environment and are not perhaps as assertive as I am. Patient care may suffer and the nurse's professional integrity may be undermined thus putting him or her at risk professionally. In my role now, I use my own experiences to inform the training and development I feel are necessary for new nurses working in prisons and to educate officers about the role, philosophy and professional accountability of qualified nurses.

This incident changed my ways of knowing, as it was one of the many incidents that prompted me to learn about organisational culture and its impact on practice. My prison experiences also prompted me to research the care/custody philosophy interface in the prison setting.

Conclusion

I hope that, as a consequence of my own reflections in this chapter, other nurses working or thinking of working in prison health care will learn from my experience as I did. The blame culture evident in that particular prison at the time of the incident discussed was quite obvious, and the effect it had on staff was noticeable. I feel that as prison health care moves closer to the NHS, the blame culture will subside as the wider world of nursing brings with it a culture of learning from experience and mistakes. It is here that I think clinical supervision in prison health care will be invaluable. Reflecting on practice through clinical supervision will give practitioners the time and space to reflect and grow in a safe and secure environment.

Prison health care is rapidly developing and becoming more accepted by the wider nursing community at a time when it is undergoing massive organisational change. At no other time in the history of prison nursing could the promotion and adoption of reflective practice be more timely. Nurses working within the service and being recruited into it are exposed to cultures and attitudes very different from the mainstream nursing philosophy. As more nurses work in this challenging environment, the use of reflective practice will not only serve to improve clinical practice but will, through effective clinical supervision, provide a supportive and dynamic environment for development.

References

Burrow, S. (1993) The role conflict of the forensic nurse. *Senior Nurse*, **13**(5): 20–5.
Chapman, C. (1980) The rights and responsibilities of nurses and patients. *Journal of Advanced Nursing*, **5**(2): 127–34.
Dale, C. and Woods, P. (2001) *Caring for Prisoners*. RCN, London.
Doyle, J. (1999) A qualitative study of factors influencing psychiatric nursing practice in Australian prisons. *Perspectives in Psychiatric Care*, **35**(1): 29–35.
Droes, N. (1994) Correctional nursing practice. *Journal of Community Health Nursing*, **11**(4): 201–10.
Freshwater, D., Walsh, L. and Storey, L. (2002a) Developing leadership through clinical supervision: part one. *Nursing Management*, **8**(8): 10–13.
Freshwater, D., Walsh, L. and Storey, L. (2002b) Developing leadership through clinical supervision: part two. *Nursing Management*, **8**(9): 16–20.

Gulotta, K. (1986) Factors affecting nursing practice in a correctional health care setting. *Journal of Prison and Jail Health*, **6**(1): 3–22.

HM Prison Service (2003) www.hmprisonservice.gov.uk (last accessed 12/9/03).

HMIP (1996) *Patient or Prisoner*. HMSO, London.

Johns, C. (1998) In *Transforming Nursing through Reflective Practice* (Johns, C. and Freshwater, D., eds), p. 4. Blackwell Science, Oxford.

NHS Executive (2000) *The NHS Plan*. Department of Health, London.

NHS Executive and HM Prison Service (1999) *The Future Organisation of Prison Health Care*. Department of Health, London.

NHS Executive and HM Prison Service (2000) *Nursing in Prison*. HMSO, London.

NHS Executive and HM Prison Service (2001) *Health Promoting Prisons: A Shared Approach*. HMSO, London.

Norman, A. and Parrish, A. (2002) *Prison Nursing*. Blackwell Science, Oxford.

Schafer, P. (1997) When a client develops an attraction: successful resolution versus boundary violation. *Journal of Psychiatric and Mental Health Nursing*, **4**: 203–11.

Stevens, R. (1993) When your clients are in jail. *Nursing Forum*, **28**(4): 4–5.

UKCC and University of Central Lancashire (1999) *Nursing in Secure Environments*. UKCC, London.

Walsh, E. (1998) Nurses' Perceptions of Working in a Male Prison. Unpublished MSc dissertation, Kings College, London.

Willcox, A. (2002) Nursing in prisons: understanding educational needs through a case study approach. *Learning in Health and Social Care*, **1**(4): 180–90.

Chapter 7

Voice as a Metaphor for Transformation through Reflection

Christopher Johns and Helen Hardy

Helen is a staff nurse working in an adolescent orthopaedic unit. Christopher is her guide within a formal guided reflection relationship that existed on an educational course dedicated to enabling practitioners from diverse backgrounds to learn through reflection on their everyday experiences. In this chapter we aim to demonstrate Helen's journey of transformation to realise desirable practice. Central to this journey is her becoming empowered to act on her emerging insights. How might empowerment be recognised and plotted along the journey? To illuminate this process we draw on Belenky *et al.*'s (1986) development of voice as a metaphor for empowerment and ultimately transformation.

Transformation is a purposeful and active process of being and becoming, of realising desirable practice as a lived reality. The idea of being active is captured by Fay (1987) who describes an *active stance* towards creating the conditions whereby one can realise desirable practice. Fay argues that an active stance compromises four fundamental dispositions towards the world: openness and curiosity, intelligence, wilfulness or commitment, and reflectiveness.

The disposition to be reflective

Fay suggests that people can only be truly reflective when the first three dispositions are in place. Hence much of what is called reflection is in fact learning these fundamental dispositions. Until these dispositions are learnt, the transformational potential of reflection will be limited.

Openness and curiosity

We must provoke the reader by suggesting that most nurses, like people everywhere, are creatures of habit. They cling to the known and familiar because it is comfortable to do so. It is also a fact that people generally learn through experience – so what worked last time is used again. In other words, practitioners are generally closed to new ideas and, as a consequence, are essentially non-reflective at least on any critical level. Curiosity suggests that we are sufficiently interested in our practice in order to pay attention to it. As such, if practice does not matter to us, why would we pay attention to it? If people are closed, they do not ask questions of the world: Why are things like this? Why do I respond as I do? Is there a better way of responding? Models of reflection may help the practitioner to develop the capacity to ask meaningful and critical questions of self and practice.

Intelligence

Fay (1987, p. 48) notes that intelligence is:

> the disposition to alter one's beliefs and ensuing behaviour on the basis of new information about the world. This can happen in one or two ways: one either gives up an old belief or acquires a new one. But both occur on the basis of new information about one's environment.

This information is gathered by gaining insights through reflection. One of the difficulties with Fay's idea of *intelligence* is that it assumes people are rational human beings. Fay recognises that people cannot respond rationally to the world for reasons of tradition, authority and embodiment. Tradition and authority relate to social forces that construct normal patterns of relating within everyday practice and which constitute the status quo. Embodiment refers to the way the self has learnt to think, feel and respond in certain ways that need to be unlearnt or transformed in order to think, feel and respond differently.

Wilfulness or commitment

Fay (1987, p. 50) describes wilfulness as 'the disposition to act on the basis of one's reflections'. Fay suggests that the practitioner can make deliberate choices as to whether to act on insights. Taking action always has consequences for better or for worse, for either the practitioner or others. Hence taking action is always a moral act to do good: an act of integrity to fulfil one's responsibility to be a caring person. Yet if we are more concerned for our own welfare than that of our patients, we may choose not to take action if we anticipate personal discomfort. Mezirow (1981, p. 7) notes that 'the traumatic severity of the disorientating dilemma (contradiction) is clearly a factor in establishing the probability of a transformation.'

The practitioner may also need a strong injection of courage or self-belief to act on insights. In Kieffer's (1984) study of empowerment of grass-roots leaders in the USA, his respondents referred with great emotional intensity to the importance of an external guide to sustain their emergence. This is probably more true where practitioners are struggling to act from situations of oppression. Nursing in our view is an example of a profession struggling to assert itself against the more powerful disciplines of management and medicine anxious to maintain the status quo and keep nurses subordinate. Alongside the external guide Kieffer's respondents also highlighted the significance of a supportive peer community, a point that is highlighted in other chapters of this book.

Reflectiveness

Fay describes reflectiveness (1987, p. 49) as:

> the disposition to evaluate one's own desires and beliefs on the basis of some such criterion as whether they are justified by the 'evidence'; whether they are mutually consistent; whether they are in accord with some ideal; or whether they provide the greatest possible satisfaction – all in aid in answering the question: 'What is the proper end of my life and thus what sort of person ought I to be?'

Fay's description of reflectiveness suggests that reflection must always be a process of ideological critique in order to 'know' desirable practice. Only with this understanding can contradiction be surfaced. Reflection is then turned towards ways in which the contradiction might be resolved. Cox *et al.* (1991, p. 387) put it succinctly:

> As we come to expose these self-imposed limitations, then the focus of our reflection shifts towards new action, towards the ways in which we might begin to reconstruct and act differently within our world's.

However, as I have suggested, exposing these *self-imposed limitations* may not be easy, simply because they are normative. Practitioners may have deluded themselves that they do understand the nature of desirable practice and act congruently with their values. Lather (1986, p. 264) terms this as false consciousness:

> The denial of how our common-sense ways of looking at the world are permeated with meanings that sustain our disempowerment.

From this perspective, reflection can be viewed as a process of coming to see ourselves truly as though windscreen wipers have cleaned the lens of perception. This process emerges from openness, curiosity, intelligence and wilfulness.

Enlightenment, empowerment and emancipation

Transformation as a process can be positioned within Fay's (1987) stages of enlightenment, empowerment and emancipation. Enlightenment is coming to an understanding of the way one feels, thinks and responds within a particular situation and appreciating the way the environment constrains the realisation of desirable practice. Only with insight can the practitioner reasonably contemplate alternative ways of responding to practice in different, more desirable ways. Empowerment is the energy to take action based on insights towards realising desirable practice. Energy is a mixture of commitment, confidence based on understanding, and the sense of conflict. It is about shedding fear, and gaining the sense of freedom to do something significant in changing one's practice or life. It is the movement from passivity toward Fay's active stance, to act with integrity and take responsibility for one's own life. Maxine Greene elegantly grasps the nature of empowerment (1988, p. 3):

To become different is not simply to will oneself to change. There is the question of being able to accomplish what one chooses to do. It is not only a matter of the capacity to choose; it is the matter of the power to act to attain one's purposes. We shall be concerned with intelligent choosing and yes, humane choosing, as we shall be with the kinds of conditions necessary for empowering persons to act on what they choose.

Emancipation is the transformation of self as a consequence of taking action whereby *more* desirable action has been realised. We emphasise *more* to acknowledge that transformation is a dynamic process of being and becoming rather than any end state.

Voice as metaphor

Belenky *et al.* (1986) interviewed women in order to appreciate their development of voice as a metaphor for their intellectual emergence. From their data Belenky *et al.* constructed five levels of voice: silence, received knowing, subjective knowing, procedural knowing and constructed knowing.

Silence

At this level women simply do not have a voice. Silence is an oppressed voice subjugated by more dominant voices, usually with a threat of sanction.

Received knowing

At the received level of voice, women conceive themselves as capable of receiving, even reproducing, knowledge from the all knowing external authorities but not capable of creating knowledge of their own. The practitioner who responds from the position of received voice inevitably views her practice in a rigid, unimaginative and narrow way. Ways of responding are prescribed rather than interpreted. Intuition is stifled and with it the necessary ability to interpret sources of knowledge creatively and imaginatively within the context of each complex clinical moment. Received knowledge is generally presented in abstract ways, and the philosophy of its construction assumes that it can explain and predict practice and so can be applied within situations without judgement. Such knowledge disassociates theory from practice as two distinct types of knowing. Yet, because received knowledge is abstract, it assumes that people can be reduced to objects to be manipulated. This is the mode of the technician: to follow and be regulated by the rules. At this level of knowing, nurses are not capable of caring.

Subjective knowing: the inner voice and quest for self

Belenky *et al.* (1986, p. 54) state that:

subjective knowing is the move away from silence and an externally oriented perspective on knowledge and truth eventuates in a new conception of truth as personal, private, and subjectively known or intuited.

In other words, subjective knowing is self-acceptance: that what the practitioner feels and thinks is significant in relation to her practice. Subjective knowing is the starting point of reflection. It is the expression and connection with self and with others. It is the connection with others that enables people to validate their voice as significant. However, it is an opinionated voice that lacks authority because it is partial and uncritical.

Procedural knowing: the separate and connected voices

There are two complementary voices within procedural knowing, the separate and connected voices. Connected knowing is connecting with the experience of another through empathy (Johns 2004). For the practitioner it evokes the question: what meaning does this health event have for the person; what does the person feel and think? To be empathic and connect with the experience of the other, the practitioner must clean the empathic lens of her own concerns in order to see the person in terms of that person's experience.

In contrast, the separate voice is dispassionate in its ability to critique and reason as it seeks to understand things in terms of logic and procedures. It is the antithesis of received knowledge. No longer is knowledge accepted on face value. Instead it is challenged for its validity and appropriateness to inform the particular situation. This voice is the dominant voice within organisations, thirsting for the 'facts' and reasoned argument, even though most decisions are made in terms of authority and subjectivity (Johns 2004).

Constructed knowing: integrating the voices into a passionate whole

Constructed knowing is the weaving of the subjective and procedural voices into an assertive, passionate and informed voice. It is the voice of wisdom, ever vigilant to ensure best practice and yet always open to possibility.

Helen's experiences

Through Helen's experiences her journey through the voices towards constructed voice structures the narrative. As we move through the narrative, we can look back to see the way Helen is transformed through the *different levels of voice that led us to the next level.*

Moving out of silence

"Initially when I reflected on experiences I recall feeling downtrodden by doctors and undervalued by other members of the multidisciplinary team. I identified a need to become more assertive. By reflecting on situations that exposed my lack of self-confidence I was able to become more in tune with my feelings. Prior to incorporating reflection into my practice, I found the easiest way to deal with conflict was to accommodate the other professional's opinions. In doing so I felt I was failing both my patients and myself. After experiencing a number of situations where doctors ignored what I had to say, my relationships with them became a focus for reflection. The difficulty I had in giving them feedback or challenging their perspective when I knew it was not in the patient's best interests was undermining my integrity and compromising my practice. I lacked confidence in entering a discussion with a doctor, and yet felt frustrated when he or she did not recognise my experience. Sharing these experiences within the guided reflection group I came to realise I needed to become skilful in creating and sustaining collaborative relationships with doctors rather than reacting against my self-oppressed state and being marginalised as 'stroppy'. Drawing on the work of Cavanagh (1991), I began to reframe situations of conflict with doctors as opportunities for collaboration whereby a mutual exchange of ideas and respect would enhance patient care. So the task I set myself was to illuminate my transformation through three experiences."

Jack

"I suspected Jack had dislocated his hip. As the incident occurred at the weekend I informed the doctor on call. I explained my concerns to him, yet he felt the leg looked in a good position. He did not know Jack at this time and I considered his observation had been insufficient. However, I did not question his judgement or knowledge of Jack. I felt even more frustrated when I subsequently discovered that Jack's hip was indeed dislocated and he would require further surgery to correct this. On reflection, I realised that I did not communicate my observations about Jack in a direct way. I hoped the doctor would have interpreted my concerns and engage in further discussion about Jack. He failed to do so and I lacked the confidence to pursue my concerns. I framed this within Stein's (1978) doctor–nurse game in which the nurse shows initiative and offers significant recommendations in such a way that the doctor can make the decision, thus minimising any threat to the doctor's dominance. Failure to play the game is 'hell to pay' and I was strongly motivated to avoid conflict, like the majority of my peers (Cavanagh 1991).

Looking back I can see this pattern developing through my professional training. I was never encouraged to speak out in the presence of doctors. I was conditioned into a subordinate role, powerless to take independent action. I realised I did not enjoy playing this game, it was just something I had become accustomed to playing. Understanding its nature was enlightening although contemplating whether I could change the game was daunting."

Roxanne

"Some months later I confronted a team of doctors about their inappropriate decision to discharge Roxanne. I was concerned the doctors were being too hasty and explained that Roxanne had only just got her brace (following a spinal fusion) and that she had not slept in it or been seen by either the physiotherapist or occupational therapist. The senior registrar turned to me with an indignant look and asked why it was taking so long to get the patient prepared for discharge. I immediately felt the conflict. I felt put down and embarrassed and felt these feelings were a consequence of not playing the doctor–nurse game. Yet I refused to be put down. I asserted (perhaps blurted out) that it was wrong to let Roxanne think she could go home when her rehabilitation had hardly begun! I realised that although being assertive (and here I might simply say 'confrontational' because I am conscious that the assertive person does not carry the emotions I was feeling at the time) is an important part of giving feedback, the strategy one employs to stimulate discussion is equally important. I did not want to be seen in any adversarial way but to be involved in the decision about Roxanne's discharge – in other words moving from a competitive mode of managing conflict to a collaborative one. Yet it takes two to tango and the registrar was not in a dancing mood. I believe they disapproved of my direct manner and sought to reassert their power by undermining me – 'hell to pay'. Chapman (1983) has highlighted how doctors use humiliation techniques to keep nurses subordinate within the status quo. Johns (1994, p. 37) states that 'despite mutual recognition by both nurses and doctors that the focus of work should be collaborative towards meeting the patient's needs, the reality is that such issues become clouded in professional concerns about power and control.'

By taking the moral high ground of patient interest I was able to challenge the power-invested interests of the doctors and help them see Roxanne as a vulnerable person rather than as some object in the bed availability quota. This experience was transformative because in the guided reflection group I could begin to acknowledge my voice and power: that I could confront and win even though I might eschew winning as desirable. It was necessary because of the lack of professional collaboration. To be heard I had to shout, otherwise my timorous voice would be discounted.

Many of my peers within the group related to these stories with their own similar stories. The group supervisor posed the question, 'How is it, nurses, you have been socialised to have no voice in such situations? Do you (addressing all of us) perceive yourselves as subjected to medical dominance as many commentators suggest?' (Friedson 1971; Hughes 1971; Capra 1982; Buckenham & McGrath 1983; Brunning & Huffington 1985). Indeed the weight of evidence cannot deny this history, as my own lived experience and that of my colleagues testify that the issue is still alive. Why have educational processes failed to pay adequate attention to social forces that stifle nurses' voices? Is it because our teachers' voices have also been stifled? Or is it simply seen as a normative state of affairs and therefore not an issue to consider? These are vital questions to pose and ponder, for, as my experiences illuminate, a self-perceived sense of subordination and a silent voice are major barriers in my realisation of desirable practice."

Honouring my subjective voice

As my self-esteem grew, so did my desire to assert my own beliefs about practice. I began to voice my feelings and opinions. Through the process of reflection I was constantly challenged to open my eyes and view my practice more critically. I had always to justify the way I felt, thought and responded within situations. My received voice lay in tatters – even though I had been unaware of it in the way I perceived and responded to situations of conflict. The different styles of managing conflict were a reflective revelation: to position myself within the conflict management grid (Box 7.1) and critically

Box 7.1 The styles of managing conflict grid (Thomas & Kilmann 1974, cited in Cavanagh 1991)

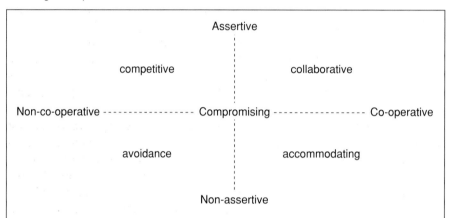

Assertiveness: the degree to which individuals satisfy their own concerns
Co-operation: the degree to which individuals attempt to satisfy the concerns of others

Accommodating
Essentially a co-operative interaction but one in which the practitioner is not assertive – prepared to give up give up their own needs for the sake of maintaining harmonious relationships and need to be accepted by others. 'Apologetic'.

Avoidance
Characterised by a negation of the issues and a rationalisation that attempts to challenge the behaviour of another as futile.

Collaboration
Involves an effort to solve problems to a mutually satisfying conclusion, a win–win situation; i.e. concerned with needs of self and others. Openly discuss issues surrounding conflict and attempt to find suitable means to resolve the conflict.

Competitive
Pursues his/her own needs at the exclusion of others – usually through open confrontation. (win–lose situations).

Compromising
Realising that in conflict situations, every party cannot be satisfied. Accepting, at times, to set aside personal needs in preference to others to resolve conflict.

analyse each of these positions and how I fitted within them. Which position did I desire and why? These are such simple yet such profound questions.

What knowledge I had been filled up with was scrutinised for its validity within each experience I shared. My assumptions were laid bare. Literally I was taught to think for myself. It gave me the confidence to express my own feelings and views about things. It was both scary and exciting.

Claire

"The issue of conflict was again central to the experience I shared in the group about Claire. She was recovering from a spinal fusion. The incident occurred during a night shift whilst I was taking my break. Claire was incorrectly moved by an inexperienced agency nurse. Claire subsequently became distressed and was crying in pain. I was upset that Claire should suffer unnecessarily and angry that the nurse had moved her when I had previously explained the need for caution during the handling of patients following spinal surgery. I felt responsible because I was Claire's named nurse and knew that she trusted me. I assumed that Claire blamed me for what had happened and tried to reassure her by promising that the nurse would not move her again. In my journal I summed up my anger with the words 'professional incompetence'.

Reflecting on this situation, I became aware that my angry response was influenced by my protective feelings towards Claire. I blamed myself for her distress. When I shared this experience with the guided reflection group, I felt challenged when I was asked how Claire felt about the incident. I didn't have an answer to the challenge, as I had not encouraged Claire to discuss her feelings. I was too wrapped up in my own anxiety. My belief that she thought I had let her down was purely speculative. Since the incident I have been 'stewing in my own juices' (Hall 1964), locked into my anger and being unable to resolve my conflict. This experience has increased my self-awareness that my emotions profoundly affect my responses to a situation. I really need to know myself better so I am better equipped to deal with such situations more appropriately. I thought I could handle conflict more easily following Roxanne's experience but this experience showed me I still have much to learn. In the group I was encouraged to reflect on my relationship with Claire and in particular my protective stance towards her and other adolescents. What type of relationship did I desire to have with adolescents?

Ramos's (1992) research into the nature of the nurse–patient relationship highlighted two impasses to developing a truly therapeutic relationship. The first impasse is concerned with power: the need to control the relationship. The second is concerned with emotions: the need to protect the patient. It seems, on reflection, that I was stuck in both impasses! And yet I felt that Claire and I had many of the characteristics that typify what Morse (1991) describes as a 'mutual connected relationship'. For example, I involved her in decisions about her care. However, I must reluctantly admit I did see her primarily in terms of her medical condition – what Morse (1991) describes as a 'therapeutic relationship' rather than as a young suffering woman. I was Claire's nurse and she was my patient, and in this incident I was primarily concerned for her safety and the repair of her spinal fusion.

Through the group dialogue, I realised I should have empathised with Claire's experience and addressed *her* needs and not merely tried to reassure her that the agency nurse would not move her again. I felt ashamed in the group that I could be so blind when the contradiction was so obvious. It was like a flash of recognition. Suddenly, and perhaps for the first time, I really felt I knew myself and the impact of myself on relationships. As Johns (2004) highlights, knowing and managing self within a relationship is a requisite for being available to the person as is knowing the person behind the patient."

Speaking with both separate and connected voices

From the perspective of connected knowing I must confess I am as guilty as the next nurse in seeing Claire in terms of my (nursing) interests, and yet I would have always described myself as empathic. Reading and discussing Belenky *et al.*'s (1986) concept of connected knowing was very revealing (and disconcerting) in light of my experience with Claire. No one said that learning through reflection was easy! I have also illuminated the way I am now framing my experiences within the context of theory, and holding that theory up for critique for its value to inform my practice. For example, I reject Morse's (1991) idea of types of relationships. From a holistic perspective there can only be connected-type relationships; the other types are merely descriptive failures of the connected relationship.

Ann

"This experience took place some months after my experience with Claire. Ann had been admitted for an arthrogram of her right hip. She was a tomboy. She hated the pop group 'Take That' whom the girls in the bed space either side of her loved, and whose latest video they were playing when Ann arrived. Immediately I sensed that Ann was uncomfortable in her new environment. In response I offered her the opportunity to move into another bed space. Ann ignored me, and her mother said, 'It takes a while for her to settle in.' Paradoxically, the mother's glib reassurance heightened my concerns. In response I decided to pursue forming a 'connected' relationship with Ann. However, when I asked her about her hip and knee pain, and how her injury had occurred, she was reluctant to talk to me. Her hobbies were football and riding her bicycle. I asked her if her pain restricted her hobbies and she replied, 'A bit.' I felt frustrated and wondered what was bothering this young person. I decided to give her some space and observe during the afternoon. When I spoke to her later that evening, she still seemed totally uninterested in me. The following morning when she was scheduled to go for her hip arthrogram she became very distressed and abusive. Clearly under that undemonstrative exterior was a frightened young woman I knew nothing about. I had rarely experienced such a negative response when trying to form a relationship with a patient. My head was buzzing with ideas about gaining her confidence. I wanted to know what she was feeling, what was bothering her and why she appeared not to like me. I felt despondent. Sharing the experience in the group I was again challenged if I was still responding to Ann as a patient and not as a young woman with a life outside the hospital. Even asking about her hobbies was related to her hip and knee injury and pain. I had also assumed that Ann would be interested in me and want to develop a relationship. Why should she? Perhaps I was just another authority figure intent on telling her what to do. As it was, she was not willing to play *my* game. The more I tried to connect with her the more she tried to evade me! Again I felt despondent: had I not learnt anything from Claire's experience? Had I embodied a way of being that defied change? The idea that *just because we come to see something differently doesn't mean we can change the way we respond* hit home.

Much of the literature about knowing the patient refers to the notion of 'clicking' (May 1991; Morse 1991; Fosbinder 1994). 'Clicking' is defined by Fosbinder as an 'immediate rapport between patient and nurse'. Morse suggests that clicking with a patient evokes the development of a deeper relationship. However, I could find little literature that discusses the relationship that does not click. Johns (1999, 2004) suggests that all relationships can be viewed along a reciprocation–resistance continuum. The intent of the practitioner is to establish a reciprocal (or connected) relationship yet, for one reason or another, either the practitioner or the patient resists this development. I felt Ann was resisting me and as a consequence I failed to get on to her wavelength, which left me feeling I had failed.

The group challenged me to consider how else I might respond. I know, from previous experiences, that disclosing aspects of my own life has enhanced a relationship. In other words I become a human being and not just a nurse. It is interesting to speculate how Ann would have responded had I done that with her. I feel it would have changed the focus of conversation away from her treatment. I felt the group gave me permission to break out of the 'nurse' mould to experiment, to be creative, to take risks, to liberate myself to be me rather than some nurse caricature. Yet there is no recipe for success. With some people such as Ann it may not be possible to develop the desired relationship. I must guard against imposing a type of relationship or thinking I have failed."

Finding my constructed voice

"The last experience I shared in the group concerned Angela. When I went to admit Angela, it struck me that I was clutching her medical notes and nursing documentation. As I sat down next to her I consciously left these files at the end of the bed and focused my attention on her as a person. The first 15 minutes of our conversation centred on Angela's journey to the hospital and her first year at university. Our discussion progressed *naturally* to the reason for her admission and how she felt about her treatment and the future. Finally I turned to the nursing documentation and decided I had obtained more information about Angela than I would have done pursuing the nursing assessment formula.

My letting go of the need to control meant that I was able to flow with the moment. I really believed that Angela and I 'clicked' and connected. When I admitted Angela the ward was not so busy as usual, giving me more time to be with her. Yet, in saying that, do I fall into a trap of justifying that time alone made this possible rather than my mind-set? Perhaps having time did create the space to be with Angela, but I can now appreciate the value of giving this 'task' more time. I can see the way we never value this talking time in the pressure to get work done, and yet knowing the person is fundamental to nursing them from a holistic perspective. All my colleagues value seeing the person as an individual and yet the contradiction between this value and ward practice is stark.

Through this experience my vision of nursing has been scrutinised and strengthened, building on the insights gained from nursing Claire and Ann. By using Belenky *et al.*'s (1986) idea of voice, I feel I have become empowered to practise more in tune with my values than previously. Before, I felt I needed to be in control and hence reduced the person to a patient to be controlled. Paradoxically, by letting go of the need to control I am more in control of myself as a person. As a consequence, I am less anxious and more creative, more able to realise desirable practice. When I speak with colleagues, I speak with a more knowledgeable, empathic and passionate voice! I hope my experiences have illustrated this journey of empowerment and transformation.

Reflection has enriched my practice and enabled me to develop new skills. It has enabled me to unlock some of the dilemmas and confront the barriers that impeded my practice. This takes an inquiring mind because a practitioner must be ready to challenge their actions and develop new ideas. I no longer feel defeated by the constraints of management and resources, nor do I view myself as a 'mere' staff nurse. I have gained an inner sense of purpose and a desire to provide effective care. The no man's land between reality and desirability has decreased as I continue to face new challenges that arise in my work."

Conclusion

Helen's compelling account describes one person's transformative journey through guided reflection structured through Belenky *et al.*'s (1986) stages of voice. The development of her 'voice' marks her passage of transformation. As Helen noted, 'as my self-esteem increased so did my desire to assert my beliefs.' It is a positive spiral of expanding consciousness. Helen has been guided to pay attention to the meaning of her practice, and challenged to realise her beliefs in everyday practice. This involves confronting contradictions and taking action to resolve them. As she comes to know and realise her beliefs as a lived reality, so her commitment is nourished and grows. She becomes more available to herself and her young patients. She becomes increasingly assertive in her 'knowing'. This knowing is now an informed and passionate knowing, informed by relevant theory that has helped her frame emerging practice issues and expand her empathic lens to see the patient's experience, yet without prescribing how she should see them. Without doubt, knowledge is central to assertion. Within the unique human–human encounter between Helen and each of her patients, Helen determines the truth of the situation as she perceives it. The 'truth' is not 'outside herself' as something to apply. As Belenky *et al.* (1986) suggest, Helen's perception is based on her empathic knowing of the other. This is the juxtaposition of knowing 'the other' and knowing 'self'. It is the synthesis of two simultaneous dialogues – of knowing 'what this experience means to the other' and 'what this experience means to me'. Or put another way, using wavelength theory (Johns 2004), the practitioner's effort is to tune into the other's wavelength. Yet, to achieve this, the practitioner must first be tuned into her own wavelength.

Such understanding illuminates the subtlety, complexity and subjectivity of the particular moment. Knowing, in response to the unfolding moment, is deeply intuitive. As such, the effective practitioner must be ever mindful of self within the unfolding moment. And, as Helen has illuminated, it is only through guided reflection that mindfulness and skilful action are nurtured.

References

Belenky, M.F., Clinchy, B.M., Goldberger, N.R. and Tarule, J.M. (1986) *Women's Ways of Knowing: the Development of Self, Voice, and Mind*. Basic Books, New York.

Brunning, H. and Huffington, C. (1985) Altered images. *Nursing Times*, **81**(31): 24–7.

Buckenham, J. and McGrath, G. (1983) *The Social Reality of Nursing*. Adis, Sydney.

Capra, F. (1982) *The Turning Point: Society and the Rising Culture*. Fontana, London.

Cavanagh, S. (1991) The conflict management style of staff nurses and managers. *Journal of Advanced Nursing*, **16**: 1254–60.

Chapman, G.E. (1983) Ritual and rational action. *Journal of Advanced Nursing*, **8**: 13–20.

Cox, H., Hickson, P. and Taylor, B. (1991) Exploring reflection: knowing and constructing practice. In *Towards a Discipline of Nursing* (Gray, G. & Pratt, R., eds), pp. 373–90. Churchill Livingstone, Melbourne.

Fay, B. (1987) *Critical Social Science*. Polity Press, Cambridge.

Fosbinder, D. (1994) Patient perceptions of nursing care: an emerging theory of interpersonal competence. *Journal of Advanced Nursing*, **20**: 1085–93.

Friedson, E. (1971) *Professional Dominance*. Aldine Atherton, Chicago.

Greene, M. (1988) *The Dialectic of Freedom*. Teachers College Press, Columbia University, New York.

Hall, L. (1964) Nursing – what is it? *Canadian Nurse*, **60**(2): 150–4.

Hughes, E. (1971) *The Sociological Eye: Selected Papers*. Aldine Atherton, Chicago.

Johns, C. (1994) Constructing the Burford NDU model: In *The Burford NDU Model: Caring in Practice* (Johns, C., ed.), pp. 20–58. Blackwell Science, Oxford.

Johns, C. (1999) Caring connections: knowing self within caring relationships through reflection. *International Journal for Human Caring*, **3**(2): 31–8.

Johns, C. (2004) *Becoming a Reflective Practitioner*, 2nd edn. Blackwell Publishing, Oxford.

Kieffer, C. (1984) Citizen empowerment: a developmental perspective. *Prevention in Human Services*, **84**(3): 9–36.

Lather, P. (1986) Research as praxis. *Harvard Educational Review*, **56**(3): 257–77.

May, C. (1991) Affective neutrality and involvement in nurse–patient relationships: perceptions of appropriate behaviour amongst nurses in acute medical and surgical wards. *Journal of Advanced Nursing*, **26**: 2–8.

Mezirow, J. (1981) A critical theory of adult learning and education. *Adult Education*, **32**: 3–24.

Morse, J. (1991) Negotiating commitment and involvement in the nurse–patient relationship. *Journal of Advanced Nursing*, **16**: 552–8.

Ramos, M. (1992) The nurse-patient relationship: themes and variations. *Journal of Advanced Nursing*, **17**: 496–506.

Stein, L. (1978) The doctor–nurse game. In *Readings in the Sociology of Nursing* (Dingwall, R. & McIntosh, J., eds), pp. 108–17. Churchill Livingstone, Edinburgh.

Chapter 8

Reflexivity and Intersubjectivity in Clinical Supervision: On the Value of Not-knowing

Dawn Freshwater

The concept of an 'interactive field' or 'third area' in the therapeutic alliance is not a new one and has been explored by several writers from a variety of differing perspectives (Jung 1951; Winnicott 1971; Hall 1984; Hillman 1994; Schwartz-Salant 1994, 1998). Recent works demonstrate an increasing interest in the exploration of 'field phenomena' between nurse/therapist and patient. There is, however, very little written regarding the manifestation of 'the field' in, and its relationship to, the supervisory relationship. It is not uncommon to read about the parallel processes that occur across the therapist/patient–supervisor/supervisee relationship, but it would seem that the transfer of 'field phenomena' both to and from supervision has not yet been examined in any detail.

This chapter aims to explore the concept of the interactive field more fully with particular emphasis on the synergy of the supervisory relationship. The early part of the discussion centres on an exposition of the historical development of the 'interactive field', including some discussion concerning the difficulties of defining the term itself. The two main vantage points from which the interactive field is viewed are the archetypal and psychodynamic schools of psychological thought. The chapter then goes on to explore the nature of and the approaches and attitudes to the supervisory situation. The concluding discussion focuses on the manifestation of 'field phenomena' within supervision and the willingness of the supervisor/supervisee to sacrifice their 'knowing' (Schwartz-Salant 1994) and to be with what Keats termed 'negative capability' (Casement 1985). During the course of this chapter, I will be referring to both the nurse and the therapist. For the purposes of this discussion I will use them interchangeably, based on the argument that reflective practitioners are engaged in the therapeutic use of self in everyday practice (Freshwater 2002).

The interactive field and the therapeutic alliance

Many authors describe the therapeutic relationship as one of two people sharing a common humanity (Fordham 1957, cited in Sedgewick 1994; Jacoby

1984; Jacobs 1988). It is this common humanity that unites the patient and nurse/therapist as equals. At the beginning of any caring relationship, large parts of the carer's personality are sucked into the personality of the patient and vice versa (Symington 1986). Symington (1986) comments that, when these two people meet, there is what he calls a 'fusion' and a new world being is created. Here he is discussing the psychoanalytic notions of transference and counter-transference. Not only does the patient draw the nurse into his personality (transference) but also in reverse the nurse draws the patient into their own personality structure. Without this fusion, the feelings and behaviours that a nurse experiences in relation to the patient (counter-transference) would not occur. Rolfe *et al.* (2001, p. 85) define transference as that which occurs 'when patients express feelings toward the practitioner they originally felt for parents or significant others'. Counter-transference occurs when 'the practitioner carries feelings consciously and unconsciously as a result of the relationship' (Rolfe *et al.* 2001, p. 85). Fordham 1957 (cited in Sedgwick 1994), however, has defined counter-transference as almost any unconscious behaviour of the practitioner, and suggests that all therapeutic work be based on the practitioner's counter-transference responses. This seems to relate to the work of Melanie and Josephine Klein, in which the processes of introjection and projection are seen to interact within any human encounter. However, these authors specifically describe the relationship between mother and child (Klein M. 1975; Klein J. 1987).

The concepts of transference and counter-transference have been much discussed in the world of psychotherapy and psychiatric nursing (and more recently in clinical supervision and reflective practice – see Van Ooijen 2000 and Rolfe *et al.* 2001) and as such deserve further explication here. As early as 1915 Freud was marvelling at the phenomena of transference and counter-transference, finding it remarkable that the unconscious of one human being could react upon that of another without passing through the conscious. More recently Kast described her own understanding of transference, defining it as the distorted perception of a relationship in which old ways of relating are imported into the analytical relationship. In this sense transference can be seen as an unconscious acting out of the child/parent relationship.

As already identified, counter-transference is often viewed as the therapist's response or reaction to the client's transference issues (Kast 1995 cited in Stein 1995). However, the literature surrounding counter-transference and its analytic value illustrates the conglomeration of meanings and understandings attributed to this phenomenon. Sedgewick (1994) gives a comprehensive review of the more recent schools of thought regarding counter-transference, showing the complexity of thinking of such analysts as Fordham, Kahn, Ogden and Schwartz-Salant.

Classic psychoanalytic literature leads us to believe that counter-transference responses from the therapist are not productive and are potentially damaging to the patient's development. Freud viewed counter-transference as a danger to be avoided or negotiated through self-analysis (Jacoby 1984) (self-analysis is also one of the fundamental principles of reflective practice: Todd made reference to this in Chapter 4 of this book). If we were to take this view within Fordham's framework, either the therapist would be causing more harm than good or they would need to be conspicuous by their absence. The analyst may become the perfect neutral object, taking what Jung (1951) described as the 'clean hands' approach and maintaining the smokescreen of professional authority. Taking this stance the therapist may ask themselves questions regarding the location of pathology, that is, whose pathology is whose, resulting in an either/or approach. Although the idea of 'clean hands' and therapist/practitioner constant self-examination are of importance, the revolution in thinking regarding counter-transference persuades us that there is another dimension deserving attention, that of the 'wounded healer' (Sedgewick 1994) and the notion of being infected by and infecting the patient (Schwartz-Salant 1994, 1998). Heimann (1950 cited in Symington 1986), in her paper on counter-transference, actively invited rather than discouraged therapists to use their own feelings in clinical work. In this way the healing work becomes a true joint venture for which both partners are responsible. It is the idea of the therapeutic alliance as a joint venture which connects it with the interactive field.

Many reflective practitioners will recognise themselves in the above description, that is, they have surrendered the 'clean hands' approach to patient care, and using a reflective framework engage in a subjective analysis of themselves and their practices. Models of reflection actively encourage the practitioner to use their emotions and feelings as the internal compass by which to navigate their way through the daily challenges of clinical practice. There is now largely an acceptance that nurses themselves are human and as such are 'wounded healers'. This may sound trite, but it is only two decades ago that definitive research undertaken by Isobel Menzies (1988) highlighted the ritualised repression of emotions that nursing staff employ in order to survive the emotional labour of caring. Moreover, I remember one of the key messages that I learnt during my own basic training was that of not getting involved with the patient and their family. Fortunately, the self has been rehabilitated back into clinical nursing practice, with the result that practice is less sanitised and nurses are more embodied (Freshwater 2002). However, this is not the end of the story, for the inclusion of self and the acceptance of subjectivity are only part of the process, a step towards relational caring and towards intersubjectivity and the interactive field.

Personal reflections on the objective/subjective split

"As strongly as Freud cautioned against counter-transference, with equal resolution he advocated that transference would and should be allowed to develop in the process of analysis (cited in Symington 1986). Rather than seeing these two concepts as separate entities, Jung (1951) saw them as part of the interaction between two people, suggesting that the analyst could be affected by the patient's unconscious. This is something that I myself have become conscious of in my own work and have used in a traditional psychoanalytical way either through interpretation or holding back my 'self'. I am not sure whether I was trying to protect the patient from me or myself from the patient. I have not always been sure of how or why I have made this objective/subjective distinction, except for asking myself 'Who is this for? Who does this belong to, the patient or me?' I had not considered that it might belong to both of us, least of all that it might even be useful to both of us if it were made explicit. In this way I have treated both myself and the patient as objects, leaving little space for anything other than the two of us and now I question whether I even allowed that. In later years I found myself feeling completely disconnected from my work and therein my patients, and found the traditional analytic frame constraining and restricting of the patients' own healing potential and of my own creativity and imagination, my deeper self. At some level I was becoming disillusioned with my work, as it became more and more devoid of meaning.

On reflection the frame (or the way I interpreted the frame) was too tight. Although I have truly aimed to make the unconscious conscious and apportion the baggage accordingly, boundaries, supervision and personal therapy figuring highly on the agenda, I feel I lost all sense of wonder and awe at the unconscious's ability to direct us in the process of individuation. I felt the sense of wonder as I read Freud's first words on the unconscious, but somehow felt that I, like Freud, fell into a trap of trying to literalise and concretise something that was in the imaginal realm. The prime mover in this aspect of human behaviour seems to me to be the 'ego'. The ego has the desire to know, wants predictability, and wishes to move into and to colonise the unconscious. The ego views the therapeutic alliance from the heroic stance and thus aims to diagnose (find the cause rather than seeing through), administer treatment (remove, reverse, bypass, etc.) and return to the status quo (cure). Hence from the heroic standpoint, transference and counter-transference become something to be diagnosed, worked through and resolved. This seems to concur with the traditional scientific views on medicine and research. This polarises the therapeutic alliance, placing the therapist firmly in the seat of healer and the patient in the sick role (Guggenbahl-Craig 1971).

As I write this I am aware of issues to do with control and letting go and I think this is what the myth of Chiron (wounded healer) is asking us to do. This involves a transition from one realm to another, beyond the struggle of yours or mine from the known to the unknown, from above to below and a letting go of the ego, a metaphorical death. Schwartz-Salant (1994) terms this the sacrifice of knowing. Keats (1817 cited in Casement 1985) termed this, rather poetically, 'negative capability'. That is, 'when a man is capable of being in uncertainties, mysteries, doubts, without any irritable reaching after fact and reason' (p. 223). The psychodynamic frame does not seem to allow for this 'not knowing' as readily as the Jungian/archetypal frame which allows the creativity of the alchemical metaphor. Schwartz-Salant (1998, p. 24) articulates this as well as anyone when he writes:

> Engaging processes of the interactive field requires that the analyst does not take refuge in a scientific model of objectivity that is ultimately limited to sorting out the mutual projection of the analysand and analyst. Instead, the analyst must allow for the existence of an area of essential 'unknowing'. A subject–object merger was an essential part of the alchemical process, alchemy does not conceive of an observing ego . . .

Whilst I agree wholeheartedly with Schwartz-Salant, in my experience (although this approach is less scientific and more soul-making), unknowing is one of the more difficult tasks for the analyst to achieve and subsequently the patient (even the word 'achieve' has a heroic feel to it!). Besides which, one has to have an ego in order to experience an ego death – and to know that one is experiencing 'unknowing'."

The interactive field

At this point I would like to give a little more attention to the differing theories and definitions underpinning the notion of the interactive field itself. Authors from a variety of therapeutic backgrounds have something to contribute to this developing discussion. Casement (1985), for example, speaks of communication by impact. This he describes as a sort of primitive communication, which may be pre-verbal, often passing through the unconscious of both the patient and the therapist without entering conscious awareness. Here I refer the reader back to the previous commentary on the work of Freud and in particular the writing of Symington (1986) and the use of the word 'fusion'. Verena Kast (1995, cited in Stein 1995) also uses the notion of fusion. In an attempt to describe this fusion, Kast and others refer to the concept of the interactive field – the shared atmosphere of the relationship (sometimes referred to as the *participation mystique*). In other words the nurse and the patient are participating, engaging and communicating at a much deeper level than just the corporeal.

The concept of a field of forces has its origins in physics and usually refers to a field of magnetism or electricity. Although the field around a magnet is invisible, it exerts a certain force on an object entering that field. The German-born psychologist Kurt Lewin (1952, cited in De Board 1978) developed the notion of the force field. He posited that each individual exists in a psychological field of forces that both determines and limits the individual's behaviour. Lewin called this psychological field the individual's 'life space'. In his research, from which he developed the field theory, he demonstrated how the subjective and objective elements interact in the social field. Lewin stresses the importance of individuals communicating to each other the structure of their life spaces with the object of equalising them. In the main Lewin explored the implications of his research findings for group behaviour. However, his work has been adapted and developed by many researchers, theorists and practitioners, who believe that his findings are highly relevant and have some parallels to the interactive field that is the nurse–patient relationship. Consider, for example, the wealth of literature that builds on the concept of action research and action learning, and the impact that this literature has had on that of reflection and reflective practice (and vice versa).

The question of how to communicate the structure of the life space of the therapeutic relationship is one that I experience myself as I fumble around with some of the answers, most of which are not mine. It feels as if the fusion can lead to confusion and I am left with the idea that this might be part of what happens in the field when two life spaces merge. Casement (1985) seems to be considering this type of communication and its application to the analytic field when he writes on projective identification. He draws upon the work of Winnicott, stating that, in order for the analyst to feel the full impact of the patient's projections, there needs to be a space, a period of suspended attention. This I take to mean yielding to the not knowing, allowing room for 'reverie' (Bion 1974) or what Winnicott (1971) preferred to call the 'play space', and what Keats (Casement 1985) may have meant by negative capability.

Most writers seem to agree that in the initial phases of the therapeutic alliance it is important for the therapist to be able to contain both themselves and the patient and their projections. I would argue that this early phase of the relationship is essential to the subsequent revelation of the field phenomena. It seems a tautology to state that, for two separate subjects to merge, there first needs to be a notion of two separate subjects. Here I am saying that the ability of the practitioner to build and create a safe container for their patient and themselves to work within will have a subsequent effect on whether or not the dyad will feel able to surrender to the interactive field. Although I have used the word 'container' as used by Casement (1985), I could just as easily use the term 'holding environment' (Winnicott 1971) or 'temenos' (vessel: Jung 1951).

If my projections are in the field, the patient is just as likely to be magnetically attracted to them as I to his. We become entwined in each other's space knowingly and unknowingly. How would it be if my projections and the patient's projections were combined and we both got inside them? What would be our subjective experience of this created third – what would be the impact of the third, the collective, on the two?

Schwartz-Salant (1994) suggests that the only way for the therapist to fully experience the inhabitants of the interactive field is to move house, i.e. to move into the field themselves. The field cannot be illuminated by conscious interpretation; it is a place of mystery where explanations destroy symbolic meaning. The interactive field needs to become the focus of observation in order that it can become 'a presence that both people are inside of and simultaneously, observers of' (Schwartz-Salant 1994, p. 5). Thus the nurse and the patient are revealing their own humanness, with all its frailties, complexities and wounds. This has challenged and continues to challenge the traditional psychoanalytic notion of what constitutes a therapeutic relationship.

Personal reflections on the interactive field

It is so difficult to talk of the interactive field through ego language, but equally it seems just as hard to discuss the notion of surrendering to an interactive field unless one is coming from a place of ego boundary and strength. I feel that the boundaries of the personal consciousness do have to have some shape in order that the person feels that they have something to come back to if they let go. I also muse on the thought that the interactive field could become an ego-centred technique in therapy, in other words the ego could just as easily become attached to not-knowing as it was to knowing. For me it is a simple case of saying, 'You can't get in the bath with your patient if one hasn't been created.' This will depend upon the individual relationship that is developed with each individual patient. I would like to share a personal experience of this shift from being outside the field to being contained by the field. This experience came after 41 sessions of intense work with this particular patient, who will be referred to here as Ann. I will give a brief synopsis of Ann's history by way of introduction.

Ann

"Ann is aged 42 years and works as a carer in a psychiatric day centre. She started her own psychotherapy training some years ago but had to give this up due to lack of time, finance and a relationship problem. She was referred to me via the Employee Assistance Programme as she was experiencing difficulties in her working relations, specifically with her manager. Ann has three sons aged 23, 18 and 15. She separated from their father four years ago but is still in contact with him. She has problems managing the boys and each of them has been involved in a series of petty crimes. Ann herself was one of five children and always felt that her parents were never really there. Her main source of relationship in her early years was through her daydreams.

Initially I did not like Ann. She presented as an ageing hippie and was often non-committal during our sessions. She would often drift off and I would find myself trying to ground her, although I would frequently find myself in the grip of oceanic feelings. It was all I could do at this point to hold Ann's feelings. She would very often be late and occasionally forget to turn up, and it fell to me to constantly and firmly reiterate the boundaries. My first hypotheses centred around the pre-ego and trans-ego thresholds (see Figure 8.1) and I was aware of midlife issues starting to surface. I was often confused as to whether we were working at a pre-ego level, and what I was experiencing with Ann was a symbiotic state or perhaps we were working at a trans-ego level and what I was holding were the feelings of a mystical oneness. On reflection I can see that I was stuck into an either/or way of viewing our work together, as opposed to a both/and. The more

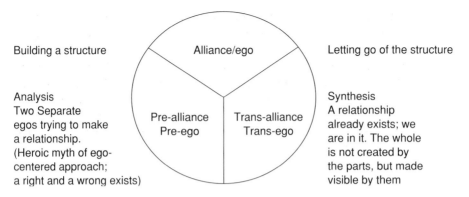

Figure 8.1   The therapeutic relationship (adapted from Freshwater & Robertson 2003)

I experienced this confusion the more I tried to sort out what it was. I did this by imposing very strict boundaries and trying to be very clear about where I was in this relationship. As time has gone on and Ann has started to reintegrate some of her feelings I have taken a real liking to her and have a lot of respect for her. She now turns up on time and respects the boundaries (and implicitly her therapist). There has started to be a mutual relationship and then . . .

In session 41 Ann leaves it until the last few minutes to tell me that she had a dream. In the dream Ann is fed up with suffering and wants to end it all. In the dream the feeling is so strong that she takes some pills. Having taken the pills she becomes concerned that she may not have completed all her business – she did not want to leave unfinished business. In her dream along comes a child who embodies Ann and her three sons, Ann becomes very upset in the dream that she has decided to leave, but the suffering is such that she has to go and she dies in the dream just as she is waking up. As it was the end of the session we did not have time to discuss the dream.

That night I dreamt exactly the same dream as Ann. It definitely was Ann's dream and she was acting in it exactly as she had said. I don't know how, but I knew in the dream that I was dreaming Ann's dream and that it was also my dream; it was a very deep level of knowing. In my dream of Ann's dream, I knew exactly what it meant and how to make sense of it. When I awoke, although I knew what the dream meant I could not articulate it; it was beyond words. The purpose of relaying this story here is not to analyse the content of the dream, although that would be interesting in itself, but to acknowledge that I did dream the client's dream (or the client had dreamt my dream). Whilst this could be interpreted in all manner of ways, at the time I chose to interpret it as my being too involved with the patient. This perspective is still bound in whether or not I was inside or outside the relationship with Ann. Hall (1984) writes of this experience when he says: 'When the analyst dreams of a patient, it is most important for the analyst to understand if he has made distortions of the patient, perhaps overvaluing or undervaluing the analysand' (p. 39). However, I did not feel that the dream could be interpreted as a counter-transference dream: the dream was not different from Ann's, it was Ann's. In supervision I was able to explore how this experience related to the interactive field in which both Ann's and my own experience are entwined. Further, it was us who were being created out of the dream, rather than we two creating the dreams. Perhaps this was the relationship that Ann and I had always had: it was only now being revealed to us through a synergy. I chose not to share my experience with Ann but I did see it as a message regarding the strength and depth of our developing relationship."

Supervision

Supervision is an established part of practice within helping disciplines. Indeed it is part of an already established norm that nurses and therapists should continue to be supervised throughout their working life (Freshwater 2003). For an historical account of the development of clinical supervision and its integration into nursing, readers are referred to authors such as Van Ooijen (2000), Rolfe *et al.* (2001) and Freshwater (2003), and other chapters in this book.

In 1980 Hess suggested that supervision should be based on a relationship where the general goal is to help the supervisee to become more effective, that is, to develop therapeutic competence. Little has changed with regard to this, although in nursing the primary aim of supervision might be deemed to be related to the protection of clients. However, it is also recognised as vital for the continued support and development of the practitioner. Exploration through critical reflection in the safe environment of supervision can facilitate insight and self-awareness linked to the process of learning. Some authors emphasise the importance of technical knowledge in supervision in relation to the development of clinical competence in the supervisee; this of course is an area of concern both for the supervisor and supervisee. However, like therapeutic work itself, the emphasis on technique and clinical competence in supervision could put the supervisor into the role of the expert, the knowledgeable one (the well one) with the supervisee in the role of the novice, the learner (the sick one). And at some level there may be an element of this really being the case, as there is in the nurse/patient situation.

There is, however, a further area that deserves attention within supervision: what Holloway (1995, p. 1) terms 'the untold area of artistry in practice'. This refers to a different type of knowledge. Building upon Schön's (1983) work, *The Reflective Practitioner*, this type of knowledge is believed to be embedded in the everyday world of practice and considers the practitioner to be the holder of the key to their own artistry. This obviously has implications for the agenda of supervision. I refer here not only to the power issues inherent within the approach to supervision, but also to the issue of who is setting the agenda and whether this emphasises product or process.

In exploring the process of supervision, pertinent questions can be asked around the dynamics of the relationship. One question that is often addressed implicitly is who the supervision is for: the patient, the practitioner, the organisation, the system, the agency, the training course? The more significant question is how these different agendas affect the supervisory relationship (Jacobs 1996).

Parallel process in supervision

The literature demonstrates a great interest in what is frequently called the 'parallel process' in supervision, whereby it is conceived that the dynamics of the therapeutic alliance can be replicated in the supervisory relationship. Here, the relationship between nurse/patient–supervisor/supervisee is accentuated and becomes the dynamic element of supervision. According to Holloway (1995, p. 41): 'The structure and character of the relationship embody all other factors and in turn all other factors are influenced by the relationship.' This seems to have some similarities to the notion of the interactive field that has been discussed previously, and perhaps the word 'relationship' could be tentatively substituted for 'field', with 'structure' and 'character' symbolising the container that is created. In other words the container is all important to the development of the relationship.

Whilst it is not the premise of this chapter that all supervisory relationships can and should be interpreted in terms of the parallel process, the similarities between the nurse/patient and supervisor/supervisee relationship are many. Both are ideally characterised by closeness, collaboration and a degree of intimacy (Page & Wosket 1994). Feelings, thoughts and behaviours experienced by therapists in their relationships with patients may be unconsciously brought into the supervisory relationship. Holloway (1995) quotes Miller who embraces the idea of relationship and communication influencing development. Miller (1976 cited in Holloway 1995, p. 15) states that understanding the relationship is understanding the process because there is:

> a symbiotic relationship between communication and relational development. Communication influences relational development, and in turn (or simultaneously), relational development influences the nature of the communication between parties to the relationship.

In order for the supervisory relationship to be one of mutuality, the supervisor needs to be open to being infected and affected by the supervisee, but as in the therapeutic alliance this does not happen consciously from the onset. However, the area of mutual woundedness may become more explicit as the relationship develops. Like the therapeutic relationship, the supervision relationship can be divided into three phases. Holloway (1995) describes the three phases of the supervisory relationship as follows.

Beginning phase

- clarifying relationship with supervisor
- establishing of supervision contract
- supporting teaching interventions
- developing competencies
- developing treatment plans.

Supervision provides a forum for the preservation or restoration of integrity in caring. As such, supervisors need to be people with a reasonable degree of integrity themselves. Therapists are frequently exposed to psychological threats to their integrity, which render it difficult to sustain the moral focus of the alliance. In this beginning phase (pre-ego) of supervision the supervisor can provide a safe space in which the therapist can explore their integrity and their capacity to hold the client. The beginning phase of supervision is likely to raise similar issues to that of the early phase in therapy. At first, defences are likely to be around, linked to role boundaries and control, with the supervisor being seen as the all knowing one. The move into the second phase (ego) of supervision may bring about a loss of innocence and omnipotence and some disillusionment as the supervisor loses some of their power and the supervisee becomes empowered (Hughes & Pengelly 1997). Holloway (1995) terms this the mature phase in which a sense of mutuality starts to emerge.

Mature phase

- increasing individual nature of relationship, becoming less role bound
- increasing social bonding and potential
- developing skills of case conceptualisation
- increasing self-confidence and self-efficacy in counselling
- confronting personal issues as they relate to professional performance.

The third phase is known as the terminating phase. I do not interpret this as referring to the end of the supervisory relationship, rather to the end of a particular understanding of supervision, the death of the expert, the leader. However, it is not just the responsibility of the supervisor to work towards a mutual partnership in supervision. Like the client, the supervisee has to be willing to integrate their projections on to the supervisor.

Terminating phase

- understanding connections between theory and practice in relation to particular clients
- decreasing need for direction from supervisor.

In the terminating phase (trans-ego) there is room for less polarisation in the relationship. Theory and practice become less like discrete entities and are more entwined. The supervisor and supervisee can be opened to the possibility

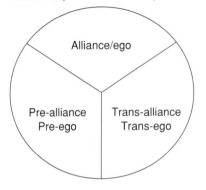

Power struggle
Role and power in supervision
Trying to discover and maintain
some independence from Supervisor

Projections onto
the Supervisor
Defensiveness and
resistance to work
being made visible
Trying to prove worth
as a therapist
Trust/mistrust
Dependence on
Supervisor

Alliance/ego

Pre-alliance
Pre-ego

Trans-alliance
Trans-ego

Risking deeper
exposure of self
and work
Beyond ego and roles
Tolerating uncertainty
Opening to the
third body
Being contained by
the interactive field

Figure 8.2 The supervisory relationship

of the transformative field. It is only when the boundaries have been clarified that the supervisee/supervisor can allow them to dis-integrate.

I have depicted a model of the three phases of the supervisory relationship based on the earlier model of the therapeutic alliance (see Figure 8.2).

The interactive field in supervision

From the previous discussion and close examination of the supervisory alliance, it can be seen that there is uncertainty at the beginning of both the therapist/patient relationship and the supervisor/supervisee situation. As the relationship evolves and a container is created, there is a period of reduced uncertainty. The early phase of uncertainty is often felt by the supervisee/patient to belong only to them, although in my own experience, both as therapist and supervisor, it belongs to both parties. However, in the process of creating the container the therapist/supervisor does not generally reveal (explicitly) their own uncertainty at this stage (and I do not think it is appropriate to do so). In the middle phase of the alliance there is a period of reduced uncertainty. However, with reduced uncertainty come control strategies, (including the illusion of knowing). These control strategies have to be given up in order to move into the third phase of the relationship, which is that of uncertainty. I believe, however, that there is a qualitative difference to the feel of uncertainty in the third phase from that of the first phase: it is experienced as mutual, the supervisor/therapist is seen to be in it, and it is less personal in that it makes room for the collective or the unknown.

Just as nurse and patient can become subject to the field in the giving up of the power and knowledge, so the supervisor and supervisee can be affected by the field in the giving up of knowing. Schwartz-Salant (1994) refers to giving up the power or knowledge about another person. In the supervision relationship this could refer both to the supervisor/supervisee and to the therapist/patient. So the supervisor gives up knowing about the supervisee (and their patient), the supervisee gives up knowing about their supervisor and their patient, and all are contained by a greater 'third body'. There is less emphasis on who is containing whom and more of a sense of being contained whilst at the same time containing.

At this stage it would seem that the supervisor is being supervised by the supervisee and vice versa: there is an object and subject fusion. This is not a blurring of boundaries (a confusion) but, as Schwartz-Salant (1994, p. 6) states:

> a state of joining can be experienced by both parties – not a fusing that blurs bound-aries, but a rhythmical process in which the field itself is felt to have its own dynamic that pulls both people toward each other but also separates them.

The supervisor can then be changed by supervision if in relationship to the supervisee; this may mean that control is given up by the ego. This is a dichotomy for a supervisor who may have an assessing role (particularly for those engaged in training supervision). Issues of power and the heroic stance abound within all therapeutic relationships (Guggenbahl-Craig 1971). Holloway (1995, p. 43) asserts that: 'Formal power, or power attributed to the position, rests with the supervisor, and in this regard, the supervisory relation-ship is a hierarchical one.' This is antithetical to the concept of the interactive field. But I wonder if there is ever such a thing as a mutual relationship both within supervision and nursing? The interactive field may be brief glimpses into moments of oneness, but I think they are just that, brief glimpses. All the more reason to pay attention so as not to miss the few opportunities that present themselves.

Whilst to some extent I have concentrated my attentions on the parallel processes involved in the therapeutic alliance, I am mindful that there is a whole spectrum of questions regarding the interactive field and supervision that remains unanswered. One point of interest is whether or not the supervisor is changed by the supervisee's patient, and, in reverse, is the patient infected/affected by the supervisor (and I am thinking more than just through indirect exposure). Is there a field that is created between supervisor and patient? Is the supervisor of significance to the field between the patient and the therapist (other than through introjection/projection)? There has been much talk about parallel process but what of cross-field phenomena? Are the supervisor's patients infected by the patients of the supervisee? I feel I have more questions than I have answers as I draw my conclusion to this piece of work. It is almost as if the closer I have become to naming the field the more elusive it has become. It will not commit itself to paper. It both wants to be known and to remain unknown. The mystery of the field and human relationship is both visible and invisible. Perhaps it is not visible in the logical and linear lens that we generally use to view the therapeutic relationship. We may only know the field as either therapist, nurse, patient or supervisor when we are without temporal and spatial constraints and open to pandimensionality, to the mystery of soul. Only then can we witness such field phenomena as clairvoyance and synchronicity, where unique human energy fields unite with their environment in an infinite domain.

Conclusion

This chapter has examined the use of a therapeutic space and has posited that there is no privileged objective position from which to view the psyche of another. The provision of a space such as in nursing/caring/therapy or supervision holds the potential to be a transitional space, a play space, one in which both parties can enter the imaginal realm of the alchemical vessel. It has been argued that for this to occur a sacrifice of knowing and interpretation is required. It has been further suggested that the process of supervision, like therapy, can be a dynamic creative imaginal experience in which both parties are transformed. And as Patrick Casement (1985) learns from his patients, the supervisee can act as supervisor to the supervisor.

A final note

I concur with Hall (1984, p. 36) when he says that:

> There is no privileged position from which one can observe (without interaction effects) the psyche of another individual. All observation (of oneself or of another) is participant observation, whether the observation is of the clinical interaction of transference/counter-transference or of the dreams of the analysand or the analyst.
>
> In this sense there is no such thing as non-participant observation.

As I have been writing and researching for this piece of work I have been paying particular attention to what has been in the field between my work and myself. I have been both object and subject and have found myself moving between being in the writing and outside it. Having re-read my work I was of a mind to change it so that I was either in or out but not both. My rationale for this was that it would flow better for the reader. Instead, I end with a comment made by my supervisor:

> The experience of the work cannot be separated from the work itself.

References

Bion, W. (1974) *Bion's Brazilian Lectures*, Vol. 2. Imago editoria, Rio de Janeiro.
Casement, P. (1985) *On Learning from the Patient*. Routledge, London.
De Board, R. (1978) *The Psychoanalysis of Organizations*. Routledge, London.
Freshwater, D. (2002) (ed.) *Therapeutic Nursing: Improving Patient Care through Reflection*. Sage, London.

Freshwater, D. (2003) *Counselling Skills for Nurses, Midwives and Health Visitors*. Open University Press, Buckingham.

Freshwater, D. and Robertson, C. (2003) *Emotions and Needs*. Open University Press, Buckingham.

Guggenbahl-Craig, A. (1971) *Power in the Helping Professions*. Spring Publications, Zurich.

Hall, J.A. (1984) *Dreams and Transference/Counter-transference: the Transformative Field*, pp. 31–51, Chiron, Wilmette, IL.

Hess, A.K. (1980) *Psychotherapy Supervision. Theory, Research and Practice*. John Wiley, New York.

Hillman, J. (1994) *The Essential James Hillman – A Blue Fire*. Routledge, London.

Holloway, E. (1995) *Clinical Supervision – A Systems Approach*. Sage, London.

Hughes, L. and Pengelly, P. (1997) *Staff Supervision in a Turbulent Environment*. Jessica Kingsley, London.

Jacobs, M. (1988) *Psychodynamic Counselling in Action*. Sage, London.

Jacobs, M. (1996) *In Search of Supervision*. Open University Press, Buckingham.

Jacoby, M. (1984) *The Analytic Encounter. Transference and Human Relationship*. Inner City Books, Toronto.

Jung, C. (1951) *Fundamental Questions of Psychotherapy*. Collected Works 16.

Klein, J. (1987) *Our Need for Others and its Roots in Infancy*. Routledge, London.

Klein, M. (1975) *The Writings of Melanie Klein*, Vol. 3. Hogarth, London.

Menzies, I.A.P. (1988) *Containing Anxiety in Institutions*. Free Association Books, London.

Page, S. and Wosket, V. (1994) *Supervising the Counsellor: A Cyclical Model*. Routledge, London.

Rolfe, G., Freshwater, D. and Jasper, M. (2001) *Critical Reflection for Nurses and the Caring Professions*. Palgrave, Basingstoke.

Schön, D.A. (1983) *Educating the Reflective Practitioner*. Jossey Bass, London.

Schwartz-Salant, N. (1994) *Transference/Countertransference. Chiron: A Review of Jungian Analysts*. Chiron, Wilmette, IL.

Schwartz-Salant, N. (1998) *The Mystery of Human Relations. Alchemy and the Transformation of Self*. Routledge, London.

Sedgewick, P. (1994) *The Wounded Healer: Countertransference from a Jungian Perspective*. Routledge, London.

Stein, M. (1995) *The Interactive Field in Analysis*. Chiron, IL.

Symington, N. (1986) *The Analytic Experience*. Free Association, London.

Van Ooijen, E. (2000) *Clinical Supervision: A Practical Guide*. Churchill Livingstone, London.

Winnicott, D.W. (1971) *Playing and Reality*. Tavistock, London.

Chapter 9

The Beast and the Star: Resolving Contradictions within Everyday Practice

Ruth Morgan and Christopher Johns

Introduction

In this chapter we present Ruth's narrative as an example of reflective writing produced as an assignment whilst undertaking a dedicated reflective practice course. As an introduction we want to briefly paint the educational background to Ruth's narrative. We are mindful that much has already been written about education and reflective practice (Rolfe *et al.* 2001; Parker 2002; Randle 2002; Wagner 2002). Whilst we do not review this literature, we do draw the interested reader's attention to it, and notably to the idea of dialogue. We ask that the reader considers how reflection might be accommodated into a professional health care curriculum in ways that best facilitate the growth of professional expertise.

In response, it is important to consider whether reflection is essentially an educational technique or relates to the learning culture itself. This consideration is fundamental because it reflects a paradigm clash between theory-led teaching and practice-led learning. As an educational technique, reflection would be used alongside other teaching techniques governed by the educationalist's agenda. As a learning culture, reflection is the core around which spin information systems to inform the process of learning through everyday experience governed by the practitioner's agenda.

The 'Becoming a reflective and effective practitioner' course (60 credits at degree level) is open to health care practitioners from diverse backgrounds. It comprises a mixture of 20 × 3-hour guided reflections interspersed with eight workshops that look at reflection from broader perspectives (Box 9.1).

In the guided reflection sessions, practitioners reflect on experiences they choose to share concerning their practice. The group emphasis is to create a community of inquiry whereby the group guide is the external enabler. Clearly, the ability of the guide to facilitate learning is essential to the success of the reflective curriculum. A guided reflection approach to developing professional expertise is appropriate for practitioners along the novice–expert continuum (Dreyfus & Dreyfus 1996). Perhaps for novice practitioners taking their first tentative steps along the discipline's complex road, guidance needs

Box 9.1   Course workshops

Workshop	Activities
Journaling	Students are encouraged to journal throughout the course as a daily activity, selecting from their journal which experiences to share within the guided reflection groups. Models of reflection are offered to guide this process.
Reflection as art × 2	Students are encouraged to explore art form as a medium for reflection on experience to open the student to access and use the 'whole brain' rather than just the 'left brain' within the largely cognitive approaches to reflection (see Chapter 1). In this way the student is liberated to imagine and be creative and use art form throughout the course, although few actually do.
Theory and philosophy of reflection	The students reflect on their first 12 weeks of becoming reflective to tease out key dynamics and frame these within theories and techniques of reflection in preparation for assignment 2.
Constructing everyday practice through reflection	The student is challenged about how she or he appreciates the patient/client/family's life-pattern and the ways such appreciation might be developed. A reflective framework such as the Burford NDU Model: Caring in Practice (Johns 1994, 2004) is used, and the significance of intuition and empathy is stressed.
Developing reflective standards of care	The student explores ways in which clinical governance can be implemented through reflective techniques, clinical supervision, clinical audit and a particular emphasis on standards of care.
Therapeutic touch	This workshop intends to increase the student's awareness of energy and the body using therapeutic touch to read the body and reflect on space.

to be more directive. As experience and knowing accumulate, there is a necessary shift to a more insight-oriented guidance that reflects a move from reliance on linear models of thinking to intuition.

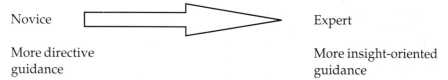

Novice   Expert

More directive   More insight-oriented
guidance   guidance

Yet either way, guidance is a soft hand, responsive to the individual practitioner's emerging experiences towards enabling him or her to realise desirable and expert practice. It is learning that is fundamentally situated in the complex, political, indeterminate, ethical swamplands of everyday practice.

Dialogue

Group learning and guidance take place through dialogue. The first art of dialogue is listening: not listening in the traditional sense, but *deep listening*. Often the experiences practitioners reveal are stories of trauma. To be truly listened to is healing.

> One of the easiest human acts is also the most healing. Listening to someone. Simply listening. Not advising or coaching, but silently and fully listening . . . Listening moves us closer; it helps us become more whole, healthier, more holy. Not listening creates fragmentation, and fragmentation always causes more suffering.
>
> (Wheatley 2002, pp. 88–90)

Wheatley's words illuminate that guided reflection is therapeutic space yet without therapising the practitioner. Perhaps health care workers forget that listening is so deeply therapeutic, wrapped up as they often are in technology or procedure. Reflection can become technique oriented whereby the practitioner feels invaded and processed. Listening is a mindful act. The group and guide listen with purpose to the stories being told. Listening is an act of connection with the experience of the other in terms of the other's perspectives. It involves clarifying what the person has said, and picking up and pursuing signs in the effort to enable the other to find meaning in their experience. In doing so the guide is mindful of suspending their own assumptions and values to hear and accept the other's perspectives. In this sense listening might be described as *hermeneutic* empathy. Heidegger (1962) explicates this as 'the essential foundations for everyday circumspective interpretation' (p. 191). He sets out a three-fold fore-structure of understanding upon which all interpretation is grounded. This consists of:

- a fore-having: we come to a situation with a practical familiarity, that is, with background practices from our world that make an interpretation possible;
- a fore-sight: because of our background we have a point of view from which we make an interpretation;
- a fore-conception: because of our background we have some expectations of what we might anticipate in an interpretation.

(Plager 1994, pp. 71–2)

The second art of dialogue is being open to the possibility of finding meaning in the text. Whilst listeners might suspend their assumptions, they are not neutral persons. The listener offers perspectives against which the practitioner can judge their own. It is not a question of right or wrong but a fusion of perspectives that transform existing perspectives into new meanings (Gadamer 1975). The third art of dialogue is the reflexive flow between experience, the temporal movement towards a more desirable future, revisiting, revisioning, and clarifying ideas within the hermeneutic spiral of being and becoming. Nothing is ever static along the creative edge. The idea of moving towards a desirable future links with the idea of surfacing, understanding and resolving contradiction between the practitioner's current reality and a desirable future. As such, dialogue has this quality of easing suffering. Thich Nhat Hanh's (2003, p. 88) words offer an inspirational message to the guide:

> Deep listening and loving speech are wonderful instruments to help us arrive at the kind of understanding we all need as a basis for appropriate action. You listen deeply for only one purpose – to allow the other person to empty his or her heart. This is already an act of relieving suffering.

The guide is a peacemaker and a role model through his or her words, wisdom and compassion, enabling the practitioner to become better equipped at dealing with conflict and resolving contradiction. As the guide deeply listens to the practitioner, so the practitioner deeply listens to self.

Through dialogue the students and guide create the learning organisation. Issues emerge and unfold revealing the mystery of clinical practice. It is exciting and creative. The practitioner comes to understand self and on this basis takes the most appropriate action towards realising desirable practice. Practitioners learn to listen and they construct a passionate, informed and assertive voice (Belenky *et al.* 1986). In doing so, the practitioner becomes wiser, more compassionate, more caring, more mindful, more skilful – indeed all the qualities fundamental to realising desirable caring practice.

If the world is essentially chaotic, then the process of learning 'chaotically' is central to realising desirable practice. So, in response, the guide resists any urge to 'fix it' for the practitioner. The guide must let go of learnt teacher mode to flow within the pattern of unfolding dialogue, to become a guiding light and resource. This is not necessarily easy for those teachers who need to control the learning environment with detailed lesson plans and objectives.

Dwelling with

Another aspect of dialogue is the idea of dwelling within the learning group. Wheatley (1999, p. 141) notes:

> When we dwell with a group or a problem, we move quietly into our senses, away from our sharpened analytical skills. Now I allow myself to pick up impressions, to notice how something feels, to sit with the group . . . and call upon my intuition. I try to encourage myself and others to look for images, words, and patterns that surface as we focus on an issue.

In dwelling with the group, the self merges with it, and thereby learning becomes a group activity. The group seeks to move beyond the cognitive into an altogether more creative realm of sensation that acknowledges and nurtures the emergence of mindful practice. This is the hallmark of reflective and effective practice: the awareness of self within the unfolding moment, ever conscious of realising desirable practice as a lived reality.

Layers of dialogue

Other layers of dialogue within guided reflection complement the dialogue between the guide and the practitioner. Each layer takes the previous layer of dialogue deeper into learning.

- The first layer of dialogue is between the practitioner and experience – a relatively naïve recall of self in relationship with others in the practice situation (perhaps written in a journal).
- The second layer of dialogue is a more objective interpretation of the experience in the effort to find meaning (perhaps using a model of reflection).
- The third layer of dialogue is between the practitioner and guide with the intention of gaining insights towards realising desirable practice (written as text or narrative).
- The fourth layer of dialogue is the juxtaposition of reflective or personal knowing with extant knowledge that could or should inform practice.

Feedback loops

Dialogue is purposeful towards appreciating and responding to the student's learning outcomes. It isn't necessary to define clearly what these are, beyond developing reflective and practice expertise. It is this purpose that gives meaning: the 'strange attractor' around which the student patterns her learning experience. The fine print of objectives would be constraining. As the module unfolds, so the student clarifies and focuses her learning effort. It is an 'unfolding' experience rather than predetermined. It is possible to discern two feedback loops at work through dialogue. The first loop is a negative one through which the student seeks feedback to confirm that her processes of learning are 'on track', thus giving a sense of order or security. The second loop is a positive loop that amplifies the creative edge and spirals the student into unfathomed realms. The positive loop seeks disequilibrium, to create the force of conflict to fuel change. Both feedback loops are essential to nurture and balance within the learning process (Wheatley 1999).

Assignments

So, how might a reflective practitioner adequately demonstrate learning through reflection in meaningful ways?

Students undertake three assignments. For Assignment 1 the student is asked to write a reflection of an experience that has been shared within the group. Assignment 2 requires the student to review self as a reflective practitioner. The assignment is designed to enable the practitioner to reflect on self-becoming a reflective practitioner, and to juxtapose this personal knowing with extant theory of reflection to construct a personal theory of being and becoming a reflective practitioner. Assignment 3 requires the student to construct a narrative that illuminates their transformative journey whilst on the course.

Ruth's narrative is an example of such an assignment. Ruth is a district nurse. Prior to the course she had no exposure to reflective practice. It was a new idea. Her narrative is compelling evidence of the efficacy of guided reflection to nurture expertise.

The beast and the star

"There was something remarkably brazen about the manner in which Heather moved to our area; something outrageous in her assumption that all services would instantly be at her 'beck and call' without a warning or even a few days' notice. Inevitably she chose a Friday afternoon.

The surgery was alerted to Heather's imminent arrival by a last-minute phone call from a 'friend'. We were told that Heather lived alone and was paralysed. She was on her way from Luton and needed the services of the district nurses. The address given was that of the local travellers' site. Somewhat alarmed I decided, as team leader of the district nurses, to contact our equivalent service in Luton for further information. Her existing nurse, Claire, turned out to be in complete ignorance of the forthcoming move despite having visited Heather that morning. The picture she painted was very negative. Heather and her family had the reputation of being uncooperative and 'difficult', so much so that the nurses always visited in pairs. Her complex needs involved the services of district nurses, social services and caring agencies once or twice daily, along with medical loans of essential equipment.

By the time we met as district nurses for our Monday morning meeting, we had received further negative reports of Heather. Trexler (1996) warns that critical communication between staff can validate, justify and reinforce difficult or deviant labels put on patients. Sadly, our discussions deteriorated into unconstructive criticism of Heather's reported behaviour. I recall that no attempt was made to understand her difficulties or her tragic situation, and she was quickly denounced as demanding and ungrateful. We had rapidly succumbed to the trap of pre-labelling a patient whom we had never met. Corley and Goren (1998) describe such stigmatising as the 'dark side of nursing', resulting in patients being marginalised and their quality of care being compromised. This was reflected in the grudging visit to Heather that was carried out by two of the team, Wendy and Elaine, after the meeting. Geographically, Heather had moved into Wendy's patch and would therefore be her responsibility. Unfortunately, the unhelpful mind-sets of the nurses that morning, together with Heather's rude, aggressive responses, proved disastrous and resulted in further negative labelling.

By Tuesday morning the team were practically in revolt. Wendy, next in seniority to me, was particularly appalled and tense. She positioned herself firmly in the 'power chair' to take charge of the meeting. I have noticed how she appears to need to be in a physically powerful position when stressed and needing to take control. The ensuing discussion was full of vitriol against Heather: 'Must get her off our list', 'Can't have this', 'Must get her sorted'.

Stories were compared about the horrors of 'gypsy' behaviour, tales that displayed judgemental attitudes and drew sweeping conclusions about physical dangers for us on their site. The travellers as a body were effectively 'etherised upon the table' by the critical analysis, and the souls of their people were left to 'evaporate into thin air' (Moore 1992, p. 29). Having no previous bad experiences of gypsies, I listened in disbelief, but I felt unable to argue with conviction. Looking back I wish I had had the courage to challenge the views being expressed. It may at least have steadied the tide of opposition sweeping Heather's way. Trexler (1996) comments that an individual from a socially oppressed or stereotyped group is more likely to be stigmatised as deviant than a similar personality from a more 'acceptable' group.

The team appeared to be whipping itself up into a frenzy with a momentum that was alarming and unnecessary. We emailed the doctors to alert them to the difficulties Heather was presenting to us in terms of our ongoing time and resources. As she was not yet registered as their patient, Wendy held out a fleeting hope that they would refuse to accept her on to their list. After all: 'Why should *we* have to do her?', asked Wendy, resentfully.

Putting this down in black and white exposes its immaturity and selfishness, an attitude we so often loftily condemn in others, especially the doctors. The action of putting pen to paper has enabled me to 'freeze the action' and recognise the hypocrisy behind the question (Street 1995, p. 151). The doctors, however, showed no interest in our difficulties and, to this day, have not asked how we are managing. Unfortunately, this lack of concern heightened our escalating resentment and demonstrated the lack of mutual support and cohesion within the surgery team. Caring behaviour and awareness of individual and collective emotion are necessary group 'norms' for strong, effective teams (Druskat & Wolff 2001).

Wendy was so disturbed by her difficult visit to Heather the previous day that on Tuesday she insisted I accompany her. This created difficulties for me because I needed to attend Peter, a dying patient, at the same time. Inwardly, I believed that any one of the junior nurses in the team could have supported Wendy and that her insistence on my attending undermined them. In the arena of the team meeting, however, I felt unable to assert my views and so I avoided open conflict in favour of an outwardly harmonious team (Johns 1992). It left me with intrapersonal conflict, however, as I struggled with the contradiction between my commitment to Peter and the louder demands of Wendy (Johns 1996). Feeling pressurised, I complied with the more powerful voice and went with Wendy to meet Heather for the first time, leaving Peter to wait. Co-operating with Wendy and negating my own wishes was an accommodating way of managing the conflict. It prevented disagreement and nurtured my own need for acceptance and approval (Cavanagh 1991). However, it left me feeling voiceless and resentful, stuck in the sterile trap of having to put others' needs before my own (Dickson 1982).

My first impression of Heather was of a very angry, truculent lady. She was obviously antagonised by Wendy who could not open her mouth without a rude, aggressive response. I had not realised Monday's visit had gone so badly wrong. I introduced myself and, in the face of silent hostility, tried a pleasant but firm approach to her care. Heather remained unremittingly disagreeable, issuing constant demands and instructions and refusing to respond to initiations of conversation. Questions about her care were met with defiance aimed directly at Wendy: 'I told you yesterday', *'You're* supposed to be the nurse', 'You never believe what I say'.

I challenged the last sentence and was told that Wendy had an attitude problem to her 'sort of people' and would not listen to her. This in fact reflected the truth and is a warning about how much of ourselves we give away. Despite now being impeccably pleasant, Wendy was clearly today in a no-win situation.

I felt I had to challenge Heather's constant stabs of hostility: 'You know we can't work together like this, don't you?'

In hindsight, I can see how this rather patronising question simply escalated her sulky, intransigent mood, and now recognise the parent/child 'game' in process. Heather was clearly in child mode, having a tantrum, in response to our critical parent position (Berne 1964; Harris 1967; Stewart & Joines 1987). Wendy at this point left the room to fetch some water. I unconsciously switched to nurturing parent role:

'What happened to you, Heather?'

'A road accident,' came the brief reply. There was silence followed by tears welling up in Heather's eyes. I felt able to put my arm briefly round her shoulders to comfort her before Wendy returned. The 'child', having found the nurturing parent, felt more comfortable and the atmosphere changed dramatically. Heather became noticeably contrite and more co-operative:

'I'm sorry, nurse, at the way I behaved. I'm not normally like that' (aimed at Wendy).

'That's all right. I'm sorry too. Let's both make a fresh start,' a conciliatory reply from Wendy, accepting her part in the hostilities.

At the time, I was staggered by Heather's complete capitulation, while Wendy, amazed, assumed I had delivered an extremely effective lecture while she was out of the room. On reflection, 'reading the riot act' would have entrenched us further in the critical parent/sulky child 'game' we had been unwittingly playing. The question about the past actually focused on Heather's situation rather than on her behaviour and helped her feel less defensive. Her response to my nurturing mother role was that of a repentant child looking for approval (Berne 1964). Harris (1967) explains that these games are played as a defence to protect individuals from the painful 'I'm not OK' position that we learn in early childhood. Underpinning the game is a child needing a parent for approval in order to feel 'OK' (Harris 1967).

An uncertain calm ensued which was instantly rocked by the arrival of two efficient social workers. They needed to carry out an assessment of Heather's needs to enable her to receive her personal care from carers. Once established, this care would relieve us of the non-nursing duties we were carrying out. Heather was resistant to matter-of-fact attempts to discuss her needs, refusing to consider any areas of difficulty for the carers. Those who are chronically sick often feel their mounting losses are misunderstood or minimalised by professionals, and, as a result, experience acute emotional isolation from them (Charmaz 1983). Perhaps Heather's defensiveness was actually the sign of a healthy spirit refusing to be crushed by the negative signals she perceived around her, signals which left her feeling discounted and devalued (Charmaz 1983).

I left the stalemate to continue my nursing calls. This long visit had put huge time pressures on a day which became additionally fraught due to Peter's death and Wendy's ongoing angst. Heather's aggressive behaviour to Wendy, and even the apology, had simply escalated the stresses and anxieties Wendy felt about visiting her. My one experience of Heather had been more positive and I instinctively wanted to be able to care for her. I felt unbalanced by the demands placed on me seemingly by everyone, and by the absence of any personal support.

The following day, Wednesday, Wendy was back in the 'power chair' for our team meeting, firing bullets of instructions. I can see now how her inability to manage Heather was driving her into bullying tactics. In terms of transactional analysis she was replaying the childhood behaviour of demanding her own way *now*, in order to feel OK (Harris 1967). She had notified our nursing manager (Jean) that we had a 'dangerous visit' on a local gypsy site that put our personal safety at risk. She directed us to back up her statements by maintaining a principle of two *trained* staff at Heather's house each day, over the next four days, while she was off duty. She refused to consider my suggestions of other combinations of staff despite the fact that it would reduce the burden on us. I suspect now that yielding to any alternative view would have risked weakening her fragile position. In the unconscious nature of game playing (Stewart & Joines 1987) I played the indulgent parent, placating the 'child' by allowing the bullying. It saddens me now to recognise the inherent weakness and low self-esteem her aggression belied: 'In the swamp of powerlessness breeds the virus of aggression' (Dickson 2000, p. 20). Understanding this at the time would have reduced the power of Wendy's behaviour and enabled me to challenge her demands more appropriately and compassionately.

Following Wednesday's meeting, Wendy and I visited Heather and the atmosphere was more relaxed than on previous visits. I was concerned that for five days now the care of Heather had monopolised two nurses for nearly two hours each time, to the detriment of other patients. Unfortunately, our time problem was not going to be resolved once the carers began their care, because Heather had made it clear that she still needed us twice daily to deal with her bowels. I noted that, despite this claim, she had refused bowel care on two out of the five days so far. I tried to explore other ways of managing her care, complying with her needs and reducing our time commitment. This was an attempt at a win/win style of interaction, seeking mutual benefit for both parties, but it deteriorated into a win/lose conflict in the face of Heather's inflexibility and my lack of options (Covey 1989). Heather appeared totally unsympathetic over our time issues and the needs of other patients; they would simply have to wait. I tried to move her from that position but recognise now that the unfortunate tone of my question alienated her further:

'How would you feel if you were left to wait while we nursed others first?'

She inevitably rejected the implication that her demands affected the care of other patients. In hindsight I loaded the cannon even more by mentioning that I had had to leave a dying man to visit her the previous day. She remained unmoved.

My attempt to appeal to Heather's better nature failed because it promoted our power and her need. Price (1996) explains that humans can reach a state of disequilibrium in response to the stress of chronic illness, making them appear non-compliant and irrational. He suggests addressing this by abandoning external goal setting and exploring instead the individual constructs and personal objectives of patients. In this way, a level playing field is drawn and the relationship is reinforced as one of equals (Price 1996). It would also have helped to pull us out of the parent/child 'game', clearly again in full swing between Heather and myself, by giving us the opportunity to rise to the position of 'adults' (Berne 1964; Harris 1967; Stewart & Joines 1987).

Our stalemate was interrupted by the arrival of Debbie, the social worker, presenting Heather with yet another critical parent figure. Heather behaved like an uncooperative child in response to Debbie's clear, assertive statements about her care. At the time, I recall admiring Debbie's no-nonsense directness, but further reading has enabled me to appreciate the likely impact of her approach on Heather who was probably made to feel like an object, a job to be performed. Thorne and Robinson (1988) highlighted the clash of perspectives between professionals and those receiving their care. They found that patients were often fraught with frozen anger, suspicion and intense vulnerability as their wishes were disregarded. Their research found that patients felt affirmed and validated by being trusted by their health professionals to direct their own illness management. In the absence of such affirmation, patients lost any naïve trust that health care providers worked in their best interest, and learnt to make their needs known in an assertive and unequivocal manner. This of course clarifies much of Heather's demanding behaviour and shines a more negative light on Debbie's approach.

Matters with Debbie were further complicated by the electricity supply being cut off, disabling the electric bed and preventing Debbie from carrying out a necessary moving and handling assessment. Without this assessment the carers, starting their care the following day, would have to leave Heather in bed. Heather, now in totally intransigent mood, flatly refused to allow Debbie to return that afternoon to carry out the task and so doomed herself to paying the price. It could be argued that, as professionals, our controlling attempts to manage Heather's care drove her into a belligerent position from which she would lose face if she backed down. The result was an unproductive lose/lose interaction in which both Debbie and Heather failed to achieve their goals due to the determination on both sides to 'stick to their guns' (Covey 1989).

I felt noticeably less anxious going to work the next day, knowing that Wendy was off duty. Tensions in the team over Heather had been monopolising every morning meeting and then bleeding forward into the remainder of the day's work and relationships. My unspoken conflict with Wendy was draining me more emotionally than the issues that created it. I also detect now a secondary desire, within myself, to 'sort out' the team in her absence! Over the following days the team willingly tried various combinations of workers (nurse, student, carers) for Heather's visits, making better use of our resources, but going against Wendy's express wishes. The success of this should have enabled me to approach Monday's meeting more positively. Instead, I felt stressed and anxious, anticipating Wendy's furious response. It seems senseless now to have gone about things in this way rather than thrashing out our differences beforehand. Analysing it, I realise that my inability to confront Wendy left me powerless against her bullying tactics and voiceless in negotiating Heather's care. I therefore took the short-term easy option of acting in Wendy's absence, exacerbating the problem by reducing Wendy's control of the situation and thereby increasing her need to bully. Struggles of 'interpersonal conflict and power relationships' (Johns 1996, p. 196) were now in play and Heather had become a pawn in the battle between us.

Wendy, again seated in the power chair, reacted to our change in tactics as predicted. The meeting prickled with antagonism in which other team members became involved, Elaine openly disagreeing with her. Wendy sought sanctuary in the role of victim, which pushed her into demanding 'child' mode:

'I can only work in this unreasonable situation if things are done *my* way' (subtext: '*I* am the one who is suffering').

This common game is one in which the 'victim' searches either for a 'persecutor' to inflict wounds and justify her rejected view of herself, or for a 'rescuer' to offer help and support her belief that 'I can't cope on my own' (Stewart & Joines 1987). Useless now to try to explore her agenda and negotiate agreement (Sebenius 2001), Wendy was too busy with self-pitying stories in an attempt to galvanise supporters. The 'game' marched on and I was forced to turn to our manager, Jean, to help us through the issues. A meeting was organised for the next day and, feeling threatened, Wendy asked me to stop Elaine attending. I refused, stating firmly that it was a team issue and we should all be there. I note now how quickly Wendy capitulates when I actually make an assertive response.

The whole team were present. We moved into a different room from our usual office and sat at a circular table with Jean taking control. The usual tirade of negative, judgemental views about travellers were expressed, mainly by Wendy but supported by Chris and Dianne. How much valuable time had we expended on such unproductive angst over recent days? Given the success of our visits to Heather in Wendy's absence, I was taken aback by the support she received from Chris and Dianne. It perhaps demonstrates the power of bullying behaviour, causing others to swing over to her side. Reflecting on this now, I realise I must adopt a different attitude to Wendy in future. Over the years I have learnt to manage her tirades by 'carrying' her until she inevitably calms down. However, as I now consider the cost to my own peace of mind and the inhibiting effect on team dynamics, I realise that the price of this strategy has become too high.

Jean, the manager, swinging between 'adult' and 'critical parent' role, batted off many of the unreasonable demands and attitudes being expressed until eventually we were able to discuss the actual management of Heather. In the light of the evidence of the last few positive visits, Wendy was forced to back down from her insistence on two *qualified* nurses for each visit and agree to double up with carers when possible. In view of the drain on our time, we decided to offer Heather visits on alternate days with check phone calls on the intervening ones. This seemed reasonable in view of the wasted visits we had already made when Heather had not wanted bowel care and had not attempted to let us know. Wendy, for no sensible reason but hanging on to a remnant of control, insisted that the weekend day should be a Saturday, even if the alternate day fell on the Sunday. Sheep-like we succumbed to her bullying and verbally agreed, knowing it could not work in practice. Furthermore, after discussion, the decision was made *not* to offer Heather any out-of-hours nursing support because of the position and 'dangers' of the site where she lived. I had not sensed any danger or threatening behaviour on my visits and felt this decision was unjust and motivated by stigmatising behaviour. Trexler (1996) finds that exclusionary reactions are common amongst nurses against those labelled as 'deviant'. I am reminded of a poignant sentence from Ron Kovic (1976, p. 99) in his autobiography *Born on the Fourth of July* as he lay imprisoned in his paralysed body, labelled by his nurses as demanding:

'I am alone again. I have been lying in Room 17 for almost a month. I am isolated here because I am a troublemaker.'

It fell to me to take the decisions of our meeting to Heather and gain her consent. As a result of the ongoing learning process of this reflection, and discussions on my university course, I have felt better equipped to communicate with both Heather and Wendy. I have become increasingly aware of the need to develop a relationship of reciprocal trust with Heather, involving the abandonment of professional decision-making and status in favour of soliciting Heather's views and perspectives (Thorne & Robinson 1988). Nowadays we talk very eloquently about 'gaining patient compliance' as a means of achieving good health care, but this has recently been challenged by Taylor (2002) who views it as a means of maintaining professional power. She recommends working towards 'concordance' in nursing where nurse and patient jointly agree goals and plans of action in an open relationship or partnership. This promotes trust between both parties, which fosters self-confidence, self-esteem and the 'achievement of wellness in chronic illness' (Thorne & Robinson 1988, p. 787).

The responsibility for Heather was gradually sliding from Wendy to me, a shift I welcomed as Wendy and Heather were unlikely to achieve any comfortable rapport. Now I had the job of approaching Heather with decisions already made about her care, hardly the spirit of open partnership discussed above. However, I endeavoured to negotiate in a collaborative manner, seeking mutually satisfying solutions to our differing views (Cavanagh 1991). It was an attempt to achieve a win/win conclusion to the conflict between Heather's demands and our resources (Cavanagh 1991). We succeeded in making compromises, both yielding in some issues and standing firm in others. I have made specific efforts to spend extra time building a relationship with Heather in order to reduce the status differential between us. Finding things in common has strengthened this: our age, the age of our children, even the highlighting of our hair on the same day! According to Walker *et al.* (2000) 'humanising' myself in this way helps to foster friendship and provide a sense of support. I felt immensely honoured and encouraged by a sudden invitation from Heather: 'Would you like to see my wedding photos?'

As a result of this reflection, I have also given considerable thought to how I can work more effectively with Wendy. She has many strengths and assets that she brings to the team, in particular her organisational skills and her genuine interest in individual group members. I have felt in the past that there have been benefits in avoiding outright confrontation with her and in 'carrying' her through stressful situations. However, the sudden insight into the insecure emotions behind her bullying caused a fundamental shift in thinking for me, as if a light had been turned on inside (Covey 1989). My own powerlessness diminished and I recognised an opening for constructive dialogue. I wonder now if she almost wants reasoning out of her 'panics'. In recent issues regarding Heather, I have made sure that I have expressed my views. The resulting discussions have not been totally harmonious but at least they have been more honest and open. I feel the whole team has benefited more from exposing the conflicts than from hiding behind an artificial façade of togetherness (Johns 1996). My change in thinking has also caused me to be more assertive in other areas of difference between us, enabling us to negotiate mutually acceptable solutions. Johns (1999) points out that collaboration does not happen automatically: it has to be created actively.

I have now recognised an amazing paradox: we have both been reinforcing each other's own weaknesses. Our different behaviours actually stem from similar roots of self-doubt. Wendy's bullying tactics and my anxiety to please have both been attempts to promote ourselves in the face of underlying poor self-esteem (Dickson 1982). My avoidance of confrontation has stemmed from a fear of losing popularity but it has also perpetuated Heather's bullying and established a vicious circle in which I have stayed approved of and Wendy has stayed powerful.

Moore (1992) discusses how to 'care for the soul' by discovering and understanding the paradoxes within human nature. He reminds us that transformative change can only come about through understanding the hidden depths of our individuality. We cannot just make ourselves what we want ourselves to be. He points us to the loathsome beast, in Greek mythology, known as 'Asterion', a name which paradoxically means 'star'. This same contradiction of ugliness and beauty is found in the profound, hidden roots of individuality. The 'beast' and the 'star' jostle within each of us:

> It is a beast, this thing that stirs in the core of our being, but it is also the star of our innermost nature. We have to care for this suffering with extreme reverence so that, in our fear and anger at the beast, we do not overlook the star.

(Moore 1992, p. 21)

As I continue to develop my practice as team leader, I now recognise that ignoring or denying the 'beast' within us is counterproductive. The beast of self-doubt and low self-esteem needs recognition and acknowledgement before any transforming change can occur. The solution lies in establishing 'norms' as a team that recognise and understand individual weaknesses, in order to uncover the shining stars which they hide. The effect of rediscovering compassion for ourselves is to renew and facilitate our love and care for others (Dickson 2000). We all benefit: each other, the patient and ourselves!

Last Sunday I visited Heather as usual, to provide nursing care. She lay very still, crumpled in the bed. For a heart-stopping moment, I wondered if she was breathing. I was reminded of the extreme fragility of her life and wondered what on earth all the conflict had been about."

References

Belenky, M.F., Clinchy, B.M., Goldberger, N.R. and Tarule, J.M. (1986) *Women's Ways of Knowing: the Development of Self, Voice, and Mind*. Basic Books, New York.

Berne, E. (1964) *Games People Play*. Penguin Books, London.

Cavanagh, S. (1991) The conflict style of staff nurses and nurse managers. *Journal of Advanced Nursing*, **16**: 1254–60.

Charmaz, K. (1983) Loss of self: a fundamental form of suffering in the chronically ill. *Sociology of Health and Illness*, **5**(2): 168–95.

Corley, M. and Goren, S. (1998) The dark side of nursing: impact of stigmatising responses on patients. *Scholarly Inquiry for Nursing Practice: An International Journal*, **12**(2): 99–121.

Covey, S. (1989) *The Seven Habits of Highly Effective People*. Fireside, New York.

Dickson, A. (1982) *A Woman in Your Own Right*. Quartet Books, London.

Dickson, A. (2000) *Trusting the Tides*. Rider, London.

Dreyfus, H. and Dreyfus, S. (1996) The relationship of theory and practice in the acquisition of skill. In *Expertise in Nursing Practice* (Benner, P., Tanner, C. & Chesla, C., eds), pp. 29–47. Springer Publishing, New York.

Druskat, V. and Wolff, S. (2001) Building the emotional intelligence of groups. *Harvard Business Review*, March: 81–90.

Gadamer, H-G. (1975) *Truth and Method*. Seabury Press, New York.

Harris, T. (1967) *I'm OK – You're OK*. Arrow Books, London.

Heidegger, M. (1962) *Being and Time* (transl. Macquarrie, J. & Robinson, E.). Harper and Row, New York.

Johns, C. (1992) Ownership and the harmonious team: barriers to developing the therapeutic nursing team in primary nursing. *Journal of Clinical Nursing*, **1**: 89–94.

Johns, C. (1994) *The Burford NDU Model: Caring in Practice*. Blackwell Science, Oxford.

Johns, C. (1996) Understanding and managing interpersonal conflict as a therapeutic nursing activity. *International Journal of Nursing Practice*, **2**: 194–200.

Johns, C. (1999) Caring connections: knowing self within caring relationships through reflection. *International Journal for Human Caring*, **3**(2): 31–8.

Johns, C. (2004) *Becoming a Reflective Practitioner*, 2nd edn. Blackwell Publishing, Oxford.

Kovic, R. (1976) *Born on the Fourth of July*. Corgi, London.

Moore, T. (1992) *Care of the Soul*. Piatkus, London.

Parker, M. (2002) Aesthetic ways in day-to-day nursing. In: *Therapeutic Nursing* (Freshwater, D. ed.). Sage, London.

Plager, K. (1994) Hermeneutic phenomenology: a methodology for family health and health promotion study in nursing. In *Interpretive Phenomenology* (Benner, P., ed.), pp. 65–84. Sage, Thousand Oaks.

Price, B. (1996) Illness careers: the chronic illness experience. *Journal of Advanced Nursing*, **24**: 275–9.

Randle, J. (2002) The shaping of moral identity and practice. *Nurse Education in Practice*, **2**: 251–6.

Rolfe, G., Freshwater, D. & Jasper, M. (2001) Critical Reflection for Nurses and the Caring Professions. Palgrave, Basingstoke.

Sebenius, J. (2001) Six habits of merely effective negotiators. *Harvard Business Review*, April: 87–95.

Stewart, I. & Joines, V. (1987) *TA Today. A New Introduction to Transactional Analysis*. Russell Press, Nottingham.

Street, A. (1995) *Nursing Replay: Researching Nursing Culture Together*. Churchill Livingstone, Melbourne.

Taylor, B. (2002) Nurse–patient partnership: rhetoric or reality? *Journal of Community Nursing*, **16**(3): 16–18.

Thich Nhat Hanh (2003) *Creating True Peace*. Rider, London.

Thorne, S. and Robinson, C. (1988) Reciprocal trust in health care relationships. *Journal of Advanced Nursing*, **13**: 782–9.

Trexler, J. (1996) Reformulation of deviance and labelling theory in nursing. *IMAGE: Journal of Nursing Scholarship*, **28**(2): 131–5.

Walker, A., Wilkes, L.M. and White, K. (2000) How do patients perceive support from nurses? *Professional Nurse*, **16**(2): 902–4.

Wheatley, M. (1999) *Leadership and the New Science: Discovering Order in a Chaotic World*. Berrett-Koehler, San Francisco.

Wheatley, M. (2002) *Turning to One Another: Simple Conversations to Restore Hope to the Future*. Berrett- Koehler, San Francisco.

Chapter 10

Using Reflection in Complementary Therapies: Critical Reflection and Pain Management

Amanda Howarth

Pain is experienced by virtually everyone but is poorly managed all round. This goes for patients experiencing postoperative pain, pain from procedures carried out in hospital, and long-standing pain problems such as back pain, chronic pancreatitis and pain related to chronic illness such as arthritis and rheumatism. As well as being a problem for those attending hospital, pain, especially that which is chronic in nature, is also a problem in the primary care setting. This chapter will concentrate on the use of reflection for describing, understanding and ultimately managing chronic pain. The ongoing nature of reflection may, it is argued, be useful for both the patient and those caring for them by helping them to understand the experience of their pain in a more holistic way. Reflection may also be useful for the management of acute pain, especially for nurses working at ward level. However, the transient and often unexpected nature of acute pain, means that reflection may not be so useful for the patients.

Before exploring how critical reflection can be used in the management of pain, I will first consider the different types of pain that people experience. This will be followed by a consideration of how critical reflection can be used by both the practitioner and the patient when managing chronic pain. I propose that critical reflection, when engaged in by both the practitioner and the patient, has a valuable role in facilitating a better understanding of the experience of chronic pain. In order to develop a deeper understanding of the role of reflection in enabling patients with chronic pain to better manage their lives, I will draw upon my experience as a specialist practitioner working in a chronic pain service.

Understanding pain

Acute pain can occur as a result of an accident or planned physical trauma such as surgery. It has an identifiable cause, can be investigated and is usually accompanied by a definite diagnosis. Once the cause of acute pain has been identified, it can be treated, the person experiencing it can be advised as to approximately how long the pain will last, and ultimately a cure will ensue and normality will be restored. This is the sort of pain that most people are used to experiencing and that most health care professionals are used to dealing with.

Chronic pain is defined by the International Association for the Study of Pain as pain that persists for longer than the time expected for healing or pain associated with progressive, non-malignant disease (International Association for the Study of Pain 1986). Often chronic pain persists long after the tissue damage that initially triggered its onset has resolved; it may present without any identified ongoing tissue damage or antecedent injury. Examples of common types of chronic pain are low back pain, pain after whiplash injuries, diabetic neuropathy and pain related to chronic diseases such as arthritis, rheumatism and multiple sclerosis.

Chronic pain serves no explicit purpose and often makes no sense to the sufferer. It is often unrelated to tissue damage and does not warn the individual of injury or disease. Overall the experience is distressing and frustrating as the pain does not respond to the usual treatments that a patient may seek that would usually provide some relief in the case of acute pain, for example analgesics, rest, taking time off work and seeking medical advice.

Often the individual cannot identify what causes the chronic pain. Investigations may be fruitless in eliciting a diagnosis and subsequently treatment does not get rid of the pain. Not knowing what is causing the pain is a major concern for patients as they often think that something sinister is going on or that they are not being told the truth. Chronic pain is difficult to treat and manage and it is impossible to put a time limit on it. Again this is a difficult issue for people to deal with. Thus, not only is chronic pain something that is difficult to control; very often it is also something that controls the patient and their lives as they seek meaning within the experience. The limitations enforced by chronic pain cause distress, and patients have to adapt and live with it rather than chasing a cure. Many health care professionals have not experienced chronic pain and only have limited experience in dealing with patients who have it. Because of this, they are often mismanaged which can lead to further distress for the individual. The effects that chronic pain can have on an individual can be wide ranging (Box 10.1). It is thus easy to see why it is such a life-changing experience that potentially has huge impact on individuals.

Box 10.1   The impact of chronic pain

Unemployment	Sleep difficulties
Financial worries	Poor concentration
Less able to do things	Preoccupied with pain
Less satisfaction	Dissatisfaction with NHS
Frustration	Uncertainty
Less contact with other	Irritability
'Not belonging'	Anger
Not 'the person I used to be'	Upset
Difficulties with relationships	Depression
Difficulties with sex life	Worry

The reported prevalence of chronic pain varies. Elliott *et al.* (1999) found the equivalent of 46.5% of the general population reporting chronic pain. In 2002 a survey of 1000 adults in the UK found that 22% experienced pain every day or most days (Pain Society website). Chronic pain accounts for 4.6 million primary care appointments per year. This is the equivalent to 793 full-time general practitioners (GPs).

Management of pain

Acute pain is a problem primarily seen in the hospital setting. The management of acute pain is the direct responsibility of the nurse looking after the patient in the hospital and requires regular assessment, evaluation and review. Most acute pain problems can be treated for their duration with analgesic medication given in the strength and format suitable to an individual and their problem. An acute pain team who will work with the patient and their nurse to ensure effective pain relief often supervises the care and management of these patients. However, even acute pain is not always managed appropriately. A report by the Royal College of Surgeons of England & the Royal College of Anaesthetists (1990) found that pain is generally poorly managed. They called for an increase in pain services, pain nurses and improved analgesia.

Chronic pain is seen in both primary and tertiary care. As it is a long-term problem, however, its management is the responsibility of the person experiencing it with support from their GP, family and carers and, in some cases, a chronic pain clinic/service. The aim of managing chronic pain is simply that – it is to manage it, not cure it. The individual is encouraged to find ways to function on a day-to-day basis despite their ongoing pain given the genuine limitations that their pain might be causing.

Researching the experience of pain

Patients with chronic pain will try many different treatments hoping to find a cure. Box 10.2 identifies some of the treatments available amongst those that patients have accessed in their quest for relief of chronic pain.

The fact that there are so many treatments that people are willing to try illustrates that we do not have any totally successful and proven treatments. If a patient has a definite diagnosis for a medical condition such as diabetes, we know that it can successfully be treated with their diet, medication or insulin depending upon the type of diabetes they have. There is no question about them having to go off and find their own alternatives. We understand diabetes, what causes it and how its effects can be reversed. With chronic pain this is not the case, and regardless of thousands of research studies we are still looking to get a better understanding of it. Ronald Melzack and Patrick Wall best explained the complex physiology of pain in the 1960s. Although their

Box 10.2   Some treatments available for use with chronic pain

Medication	Relaxation
Injections	Crystal healing
Acupuncture	Vitamins
Aromatherapy	Massage
Herbal treatment	Magnetic therapy
Chiropractic	Hydrotherapy
Osteopathy	TENS
Physiotherapy	Hypnotherapy

theory has been progressed since then, it is still in the main based on the same principles. After 40 years we are really not much further forward with our knowledge and understanding of chronic pain.

Pain is a very difficult thing to describe. Often, when asked, a patient will be unable to explain what their pain feels like. Often, too, if their pain has subsequently changed or moved, they may not be able to remember exactly what it was like or where it was. Such indecision may lead health care professionals to question the genuineness of their complaints.

When researching pain, many tools have been designed and tested to measure a patient's level of pain. It could be argued, however, that this is a fruitless task as it is impossible to actually measure pain. What one person describes as agony may be tolerable to another, and what is described as pins and needles may be described as burning by another. When a patient experiences their pain is important: chronic pain comes and goes and fluctuates in its intensity. If a patient isn't actually experiencing the pain when the practitioner sees them, then they may not be able to recall accurately how bad it really was. People's perspective of pain also changes over time. When running a transcutaneous nerve stimulation (TENS) clinic, where the small electrical stimulators used to manage pain were loaned out, I encountered diverse reports of pain. Patients were asked to score their pain at its best and at its worst on a scale of 0–10 where 0 = no pain and 10 = the worst pain imaginable (a verbal rating scale) before and after the loan of the TENS. For example, a patient may have reported that their pain was a 6 at its worst and a 2 at its best before the use of the machine. On returning to the clinic we would ask them if the machine helped. Patients would enthuse about the machine, saying how much it helped and that they wanted to continue using it. However, on repeating the verbal rating scale they reported their pain as 3 at its best and 8 at its worst – both scores higher than before even though they said the treatment had helped. There are many reasons why this may have happened. It may have been partly because patients feared that we would discharge them and not offer them further treatment if we felt they had improved a lot; although TENS can help with pain, it does not cure it. Otherwise it may have been that asking patients to think about how their pain has been previously after the experience is simply not an accurate way of assessing their pain.

The driving force behind pain clinics has historically been anaesthetists. This has led to pain being a predominantly medically dominated speciality. Previously much of the work carried out in pain clinics has been based on anecdote and the experience of clinicians often finding out treatments that they found to be successful by chance or on the advice of other clinicians. Much of the research into pain has been led and undertaken by medics. The nature of their training and the need for scientific support of evidence mean that research that has been undertaken into pain has predominantly been in the form of randomised controlled trials (RCTs). RCTs are viewed as the gold standard of research, and until recently little notice has been taken of alternative approaches. Because of the stringent requirements of RCTs, vast amounts of research have been neglected and discarded as it has been felt that it was not rigorous and valid in a traditional sense. Unfortunately this approach does not allow for the subjective nature of pain, for individuals experiencing different things at different times, and not reporting them in the same way. I would argue that a qualitative approach has a far more useful role in researching pain as it allows for people's experiences to be assessed on an individual level rather than measuring one person against the other.

Much of the work carried out by nurses in the pain clinic is based on anecdote. This is partly a result of the nature of some of the treatments under-taken and also because of the lack of research into these areas. This is especially true in the case of complementary therapies. I therefore propose that critical reflection by both the practitioner and the patient may have a valuable role in helping us to understand the effect and impact of chronic pain on individuals and their families/carers, and also the experience of carrying out and receiv-ing the treatments that may be offered to patients.

Use of critical reflection in clinical supervision

There is a wealth of literature to support the effectiveness of critical reflec-tion facilitated through the medium of clinical supervision. It is argued, for example, that clinical supervision allows individuals to develop their practice and increase their level of knowledge (Rolfe *et al.* 2001; Johns 2002). Clinical supervision can provide an excellent forum for critical reflection which allows the reflection to be taken beyond the individual, thus taking others' perceptions and interpretations into account. An appropriate relation-ship between the supervisee and supervisor is paramount (Bond & Holland 1998; Rolfe *et al.* 2001). The supervisor can be a manager, a peer, an experienced specialist, a psychologist or someone external. The basis on which supervision is undertaken needs to be appropriate also: this could be on an indi-vidual basis with a specific supervisor, or be group/peer or multidisciplinary supervision.

All NHS nurses are entitled to clinical supervision but the responsibility to ensure that this is provided and undertaken is that of the individual in conjunction with their manager (UKCC 1996). For nurses working in the field of pain management, clinical supervision can be crucial. They are often working as part of a small team or even alone, and even if part of a team they may be the only nurse.

One of the main concerns specialist practitioners may want to reflect on is their relationship with their patients and how they deal with the difficulties facing the patients they see. Individual supervision can be supported by peer supervision in groups of nurses with an interest or working in pain management. There are many pain interest groups in the UK. Some of these are regional and others national, such as the Royal College of Nursing Pain Forum. Setting time aside to discuss case studies in a group can help in reflecting on how an individual has responded to a clinical situation and how they may respond to a similar situation in the future. Sometimes admitting one's response and actions may be embarrassing and uncomfortable, so the use of anonymity may be necessary to facilitate the discussion.

For those working in pain management who have a managerial role, meeting with a group of peers working at the same level but from different disciplines may be beneficial. There may be instances where an in-depth knowledge of pain is not important but a thorough understanding of the systems being worked within will be invaluable. An example of this is the Nurse Specialist forum, where nurses from all backgrounds, from pain through to TB, to cardiac disease and HIV, meet regularly. This will provide these nurses with an opportunity to reflect on situations within the trust that may not be specific to their specialty but can be reflected on with the knowledge and support of those who have the information and/or experience of similar situations and the forum within which they occur.

Reflective writing

Reflective writing can help a practitioner to learn from their experience. It can also facilitate the learning of others (Rolfe *et al.* 2001; Johns 2002). There are many models of reflective writing that can be used and the most suitable will be down to the individual and their circumstances. My experience of reflective writing in relation to pain management has been from two perspectives: from my professional portfolio and from my research diary.

In my portfolio I write about experiences and instances of clinical contact with patients where things either went well or went not so well. Often the simple task of writing down the series of events is helpful, especially if the experience has been a bad one. Once it is written down I have something tangible to go back to, to think about and then evaluate with a view to changing circumstances/situations in the future to avoid the same thing happening again. If the experience has been a good one, then it is worth reflecting on it to see what made it good and why things happened the way they did. There are some concerns about confidentiality and portfolios, and whether or not you would want people to see what has been written. This can be addressed in two ways: by either not writing anything down you don't want to be seen, or by having a removable section that can be taken out should your portfolio be called upon for inspection or presentation at an interview.

My research diary is for my eyes only and therefore has all sorts of things included about my research, the academic experience, the processes I go through when undertaking the research and the clinical experiences with the patients. I think this can be especially useful when the research process is taking place over a prolonged period of time as experiences and events may be overlooked or forgotten with the passage of time.

Critical reflection and its use in researching pain

The RCT is often not an appropriate way of researching pain. If the professionals caring for patients with pain use critical reflection on their practice, this may provide them with some supporting material and evidence of why they do what they do and how their practice has changed to adapt to and incorporate the needs of this difficult group of patients. Case studies that have been written as part of academic courses and reflective writing undertaken by those working with chronic pain patients are a huge source of untapped information that can provide a wealth of experience.

Qualitative research that uses semi-structured interviews to guide patients through a narrative of their pain may be a way forward. Using this method the experience of pain can be explored and discussed in a way that patients may not have been able to undertake on their own. The researcher can control the interview and guide the patient to reflect on how thoughts and feelings affect their experience of pain and subsequently how these aspects can be used in the management of their pain.

Whilst supervision and reflection are crucial for supporting those working in the pain management field, and of course all practitioners, there has been little emphasis on the role of critical reflection in supporting and developing patients. As previously mentioned, many patients with chronic illness manage their own disease and illness, often with support from their relatives, carers and health care professionals. As such, this group of individuals holds a wealth of tacit knowledge, not only regarding their own pain, but also in relation to the phenomenon of chronic pain itself. It is with this in mind that I began to facilitate critical reflection with patients attending the pain management clinic.

When seeing patients in the clinical setting I facilitate reflection primarily through interview and discussion at an initial assessment appointment and at subsequent follow-up appointments. I am aiming to facilitate reflection beyond the individual with input from myself, which will be supported by other members of the multidisciplinary team. In doing so patients are encouraged to consider how the biological, psychosocial and spiritual aspects of their pain affect their life. If these issues can be identified, then we are a step closer to being able to manage them to allow the patients to fulfil as normal a life as possible. Encouraging reflection seems to motivate patients, as they feel more aware and in control of their problems. Patients need to be encouraged to reflect as it is often something that they have not been allowed or able to do in the past. Patients who attend the pain clinic have often been passed from clinic to clinic and doctor to doctor; they may have seen four or five specialists and general practitioners by the time they finally arrive in the clinic, and often they are very angry and disillusioned with the medical profession. Their experience of seeing a 'specialist' about their pain may be a 5- or 10-minute appointment where the thrust is the medic's view and the results of scans and test. There is often little interest shown in how the pain is affecting the person and how it makes them feel and think. To get patients past their anger about their previous treatment and the perceived indifference about them as an individual is often the first hurdle. Spending time and listening is paramount and often takes patients by surprise. Frequently reflecting back what they say to you helps them to realise you have heard what they have said. Once they understand that you are listening to what they have to say, then they are much more likely to be amenable to embarking on a regimen that will help them to manage their pain.

The use of critical reflection by patients

As we have already said, the presence and intensity of chronic pain can fluctuate on an hour-by-hour, day-by-day and week-by-week basis for patients. This may be because it is often related directly to their level of activity and also their psychological state. If a patient has not been doing too much, is generally feeling well and has few worries, then they are less likely to experience as much pain as someone who has been very active and is worried about their health and financial state, etc. We also find that people's pain will go up as their level of activity increases, they then rest due to the increase in pain, which eventually will cause their pain to reduce or resolve, and they will then be able to increase their level of activity again, re-starting the cycle of pain and activity. Asking someone in the clinic setting how their pain was last week or last month is not satisfactory, as it is inaccurate because their memory of the event may be at fault and other things that have happened since that may affect their recall. By getting patients to reflect on their pain on a short-term basis in between their appointments, they are more likely to provide us with an accurate picture of things. This can be in the form of a diary written on a daily basis or less frequently if appropriate. Then, when asked in clinic about how their pain has been, the patient has something that they can reflect on that is more likely to be reliable than their memory alone.

The next step with getting patients to use reflection is to allow them to critically reflect on what they have done and how this has affected their pain. This can be the key to encouraging them to manage their own pain. Pain affects many aspects of an individual's life but we also know that the things that happen to a patient because of their pain will compound their problems and potentially make their pain worse. This goes for both the physical and psychological effects of pain.

We have already mentioned patients' pain being related to their level of activity. Patients who do too much may overwork tired and stiff muscles that are not used to being used; this will cause an increase in their level of pain. The increase in pain will then cause them to rest, which will result in further stiffness and pain in the muscles and joints. Patients who do very little because of their pain will stiffen up, making them want to do less and less. They will also find that their cardiovascular fitness reduces and that they gain weight due to their inactivity. Both of these will make them want to do less and less. The key to helping patients with pain to keep active is for them to find a type and level of exercise that they can do without increasing their level of pain. Once this has been established, then it can gradually be increased in a slow and graded way to allow them to do more whilst experiencing no increase in pain. Patients should be encouraged to reflect on what they have done: what caused their pain to increase, what didn't and how long they were able to do things for. By reviewing this with a member of a pain team such as a nurse or physiotherapist, a plan can be set in place to improve their levels of activity, which has both physical and psychological benefits. By using critical reflection the patient identifies where they have been making mistakes, which they can then rectify with the help and support of the clinic.

The psychological distress caused by chronic pain can be huge and needs to be addressed to promote successful management. It is normal for the cognitive behavioural approach to be used in pain management; this focuses on adaptive changes in thoughts, feelings, beliefs and behaviour. The patient has to be an active participant, which allows them to be in some control of their treatment whilst taking responsibility for their pain management.

A person's thoughts can affect their mood and subsequently their behaviour. Therefore, if their thoughts and feelings can be adapted, it can impact directly on their behaviour and ultimately the pain and their ability to cope with it. Patients may need time to think about how their pain affects their thoughts and feelings. How do they feel about the fact that they can't do the things they did before? What do they feel they have lost because of their pain? How is that affecting what they do? Again the use of diaries and recording their thoughts and feelings in relation to what they are doing and experiencing on a day-to-day basis can be reviewed with a member of the pain clinic such as a clinical psychologist or a nurse. Patients will often find quite unexpectedly that they are doing or trying to do things that are unrealistic and the failure makes them feel worse. Their response to this is often upsetting and causes sadness and despair that may lead to them not managing on a day-to-day basis with their pain. Reflecting critically and discussing this with a health care professional can break the cycle and allow people to find more positive things about the situation that they are in.

As with clinical practitioners, writing things down can help. The use of reflective writing by patients is something that can be useful but needs to be used cautiously. If at interview a specific behaviour is of concern to me such as their level of activity or their medication intake, I will ask a patient to record what they do in the form of a diary. Asking them to score their pain at the same time can support this. On returning to the clinic, reviewing the diary and reflecting with the patient on how their actions or activities have affected their pain can be the start of finding a way of managing their pain. Caution needs to be used, however. With pain management techniques the aim is to distract patients from their pain so that it is not the centre of their life. The repetitive and often compulsive recording of pain does not allow for this. The use of diaries should therefore be restricted to short periods of time and not be encouraged in the long term.

Some patients have found that they are able to explore and describe their pain best through creative writing such as poems and short stories. Again the simple fact of writing things down seems to help. I met an Australian patient at an international conference. Her way of exploring and reflecting on her pain was through an oil painting that she had been working on for years. Her pain was depicted in an abstract form as red and black shapes/objects. Relief and pleasure was painted in yellow. Over the years the painting became bigger and bigger and the layers of oil paint thicker and thicker. Eventually she stopped painting it as she was losing some of her previous illustrations by painting over them. She moved on to reflecting on her experience of pain through mime. This developed into a short play she performed with her husband who had also been hugely affected by his wife's pain. Many patients would be unable or unwilling to undertake such activities. She was lucky in that her artistic nature allowed her to express and explore things in a way that is unique. Writing, however, is more accessible to patients, and if this is not possible due to illiteracy or the patient's unwillingness to put pen to paper, then interview and discussion may be the way forward.

Creating a reflective dialogue with John

John is a 44-year-old married man with two children aged 6 and 8. He is a steelworker working in a heavy manual job. At the weekend he enjoys spending time with his family and playing football on a Sunday morning. He usually goes out and socialises two or three nights a week at his local pub and is a member of the pub's darts team. He has had low back pain on and off for 20 years but over the past 18 months this has gradually got worse and worse. He makes repeated visits to his GP who sends him for an X-ray and tells him it is wear and tear; he is given some anti-inflammatory medication and told to take paracetamol. He is sent to see an orthopaedic surgeon who tells him his spine is crumbling and that there is no suitable surgery: he has to get on and live with it. Over the period of a few months he gets to the stage where he is off sick from work. He can't stand or sit for long periods and therefore stops going to the pub to see his friends – he is embarrassed that he can't sit still for a long time and he is always fidgeting, trying to get comfortable. After being off sick from work for a few months they send an appointment for him to see the factory's doctor as they need to know if he is going to be able to come back. This worries John as he cannot afford not to work. His wife gave up work to have the children and his is their only income. After three months his sick pay stops. He has stopped playing football as he is worried about what the surgeon said. If his spine is crumbling, playing football might make it worse and he thinks he may end up in a wheelchair. He is worried about his pain and can't see a future without it. It makes him bad tempered and he gets cross easily with his children. He is not able to do as much with them at the weekend and starts to feel as though he is not being a good dad. This makes him sad as the children are too young to understand why he can't play with them so much. He ends up doing less and less, going out infrequently and spending most of his time in the house watching the television.

Eventually his GP refers him to a pain clinic where I (a nurse), a doctor and a physiotherapist assess him. We establish that he has mechanical back pain that is stopping him from carrying out normal daily activities and subsequently this has made him low in mood, depressed and anxious about the future. We discuss this with John and decide on trying the following:

- changing his medication
- loan of a TENS machine
- physiotherapy with a specialist pain physio
- see the psychologist with a view to addressing his depression and anxiety.

John's medication is reviewed and changed; he is given stronger analgesics (co-codamol) and started on some low-dose amitriptyline, which may help with his pain and also any underlying depression. I loan him a TENS machine and he starts to see the physiotherapist who advises him on setting some goals for his level of activity and starting to do a little bit more but trying to do so without increasing his pain too much. The psychologist arranges to see him once he has tried the medication, TENS and physio.

When John returns his TENS machine he reports that it has helped. He states that he is doing more but often has to rest or stay in bed for days after he has a period of time where his level of activity has increased. When he is able to do more, he feels great but then hits rock bottom when his pain kicks back in after he has done too much. He feels as though he is on a roller coaster of activity and emotion. John says that he is not sure what makes his pain worse or why he feels so up and down. Because of this I suggest he starts to keep a written record or diary of his pain and what he does during the day for a period of 2–3 weeks.

John keeps a record of his pain during the day, scoring it out of 10, but recording it as it is happening, not in hindsight. He also writes down when he takes his medication, when he uses his TENS and what he does during the day. He also records how he feels when he does different things and when his pain is severe and when not too bad. At his review appointment we go through his diary and discuss his reflections establishing the following:

- John does not take his medication as he should. He does not take the anti-inflammatory drugs regularly; he only takes the co-codamol when his pain is really bad, and he takes the amitriptyline occasionally as it makes him sleepy the next morning.

- If John's level of pain is low, he will 'make hay while the sun shines' and enjoy being able to do things such as going to football training, playing with his children and socialising in the evenings. The following day he is usually exhausted and in a lot of pain. He describes it as 'an all or nothing situation'.

- When John's pain is bad, he spends a lot of time worrying about the future – especially whether he is able to go back to work and how they are going to manage financially. He feels his appointment with the factory's doctor is hanging over him like a death sentence as he is sure they are going to say he is not fit to stay at work and will then be laid off.

- He only uses the TENS when his pain is really bad as he finds it inconvenient to use because the wires get in the way.

John and I discuss how he could change the way that he takes his medication and use his TENS to get maximum efficacy from both in relation to maintaining the level of activity that he wants. We discuss his activity cycling as when he is well he does a lot, and later suffers the consequences both physically and psychologically. This can then be discussed with the physiotherapist who is seeing him to try to find ways to get him to a stage where he can do what he wants but without increasing his level of pain too much. He had not realised how much his ability and inability to do things was related to how he felt about things. Using the reflection as a way of exploring this allowed him to start to understand and be more willing to discuss things further with the clinical psychologist. The team's main role in the pain clinic is to address the link between thoughts and feelings and how these affect a person's ability to function.

After attending the pain clinic for eight months, John is taking his medication appropriately. He has bought his own TENS as it allows him to sit and stand for longer periods, which means he can socialise more comfortably. Regarding his activity, he is doing less than he was before but he can do it on a regular basis and it does not cause his pain to flare up so that he has to rest for long periods. He cannot play football any more but has started coaching the local under 14s football team, which he is enjoying. With support from the clinic and the hospital's occupational therapist, he has been able to return to work on a graded basis doing a less physically intensive job. It turned out that his employers were keen to keep John, as he is a hard worker with years of knowledge in their specialist area of steel making. He is now working in a more supervisory role.

Conclusion

Working with John shows how patients can use critical reflection on themselves to start to understand and get some control over their illness. John's problems were relatively simple and we did not go into detail about the effects it had on his relationships. He described his problems as 'not being able to see the wood for the trees': there was so much going on yet he couldn't see how one thing affected the other until he sat down and reflected on issues and then discussed them with the staff at the clinic.

The use of reflection by patients is something that has been done on and off for many years but is rarely described in such terms. Its use in pain management has huge potential for further development but it can also be transposed to other chronic illness where patients need to be in a position to manage their own disease to allow them to function to their maximum capacity.

From a practitioner's perspective I have found critical reflection by the patient and myself useful. Although I work as part of a multidisciplinary team, a lot of my time is spent working autonomously on a one-to-one basis with patients. Being able to critically reflect on my actions, thoughts and feelings with the support of peers and my clinical supervisor, I have been able to learn about managing certain situations. It has made me recognise how to get the most out of the time I spend with patients and how to facilitate them in helping them to take their pain problem on board and manage it themselves.

Anecdotally I have found that a patient's ability to reflect on their pain and how it is impacting upon them will escalate their journey towards managing their pain. A combination of their reflection and mine has gradually allowed me to develop clinically and improve my skills and the way I interview and manage patients. Without the use of reflection I would have still been asking the same questions in the same way that I was years ago when I first started in this role. This would have been both boring for me and limiting for the patients, as it would not allow them to explore and develop their knowledge and understanding of the experience of chronic pain.

References

Bond, M. and Holland, S. (1998) *Skills of Clinical Supervision for Nurses*. Open University Press, Buckingham.

Elliot, A.M., Smith, B.H., Penny, K.I., Cairns-Smith, W. and Chambers, W.A. (1999) The epidemiology of chronic pain in the community. *Lancet*, **354**: 1248–52.

International Association for the Study of Pain (1986) *Classification of Chronic Pain*. Pain supplement 3. S1–S226.

Johns, C. (2002) *Guided Reflection: Advancing Practice*. Blackwell Publishing, Oxford.

Pain Society website www.painsoc.org. Last accessed 22/11/04.

Rolfe, G., Freshwater, D. and Jasper, M. (2001) *Critical Reflection for Nurses and the Caring Professions: a User's Guide*. Palgrave, Basingstoke.

Royal College of Surgeons of England and Royal College of Anaethetists (1990) *Report of the Working Party on Pain after Surgery*. RCS/RCA, London.

United Kingdom Central Council for Nurses, Midwives and Health Professionals (1996) *Position Statement on Clinical Supervision*. UKCC, London.

Chapter 11

Creating Sacred Space: A Journey to the Soul

Eleanor Gully

Some years ago I was asked to give thought to the philosophy of my nursing practice. I found this process to be both difficult and onerous. How do I articulate what I do; how do I express what is, in essence, the very core of my being within the context of my practice? After writing several entries in my journal and engaging in mindful meditation, I found myself re-reading *the Prophet* by Kahlil Gibran (1973). His words resonated within me: *You have given me my deeper thirsting after life*. Each experience I have had in my life and my work as a nurse has been food for thought and quiet contemplation. Some experiences speak more fully than others and have created my being; perhaps these experiences give insight and understanding to the person I am today. I would like to share with you, the reader, three stories which I believe bridge the gap between my inner and outer world and express the philosophy of my practice as I see it today.

I begin this chapter with a piece of poetry that for me gives witness to this reflective philosophy.

In this moment

I feel I have always been a nurse
what a nurse is I have difficulty
   defining
is it what I feel what I do?
what makes me different from a
   social worker
a child care minder, a mother?

Was nurse indelibly imprinted on
   my brain
was my DNA programmed for
   nursing?
Did I have a choice?
or did I make the choice to nurse.
Why am I located in this awesome
   work

what is my purpose in life what is
   my goal?

When I look into the eyes, the
   windows of the soul of the other
I care for and we connect
I know I have arrived
the response from the other reflects
   this wordless connection
We are here
We have arrived
two souls meet if but for a fleeting
   moment
two souls destined to meet in the
   moment
and in the moment there is change

I change the other changes
for we have met
a meeting beyond the physical, the
    tangible
a meeting spiritual and
    transcending
for two souls have touched
have shared compassion
have touched the universal
    pulse
Of a shared humanity
What is my purpose?
What is my goal?
It is to create a compassionate
    feminine face of love and trust
in a world where the dis-eased
    body is viewed through a
    microscope
separated from the life source of the
    one whose heart beats
where the broken spirit captive in
    its own world is set apart
is less than
where the vibrant soul of another
    is caught in the prison of a
    body
that is named dis-abled
Compassion is more than a word
It is the living of a life that is shared
    with all
in joy and pain
in grief and happiness
This is my purpose this is my
    goal
I feel I have always been a nurse
It is the going within my soul
the spiritual reflection of who
    I am
I am the Koru, the Spiral
I dance within to make meaning of
    the dance without
a constant movement
fluid and circular
within to feed my soul
without to meet the other, to touch
    the other

In the moment,
Moving within to reflect on that
    touch that gaze
the mystic dream
Contemplating, reflecting
giving the next encounter deeper
    meaning
spiritual energy shared.
Perhaps a seed is planted within
    both of us
where a smile nourishes, feeds its
    growth
where tears slake the seed's thirst.
where the salt of the tears heals
Where the hand of friendship is
    offered
Companions on the journey
where laughter revives lifting the
    spirits
bringing light and new meaning.
Where the creative imagination
of the soul is restored.
Moments special moments
nothing extraordinary
when my heart opens and sees
    beyond the physical
and is filled with unconditional love
barriers are dissolved, souls open,
    fear is dispelled
if but momentarily and
awe and joy flow through me,
    offering warmth and fulfilment
This gift of the moment is boundless
    and intangible
And a gentle sigh heaves in my
    breast
with the beat of my heart to remind
    me
of a common bond shared
defying race, creed, colour, gender,
    political persuasion
I know when I turn my back on
    another
I turn my back on myself
When I judge another I judge
    myself

when I withhold forgiveness or
  love
I love myself less; forgive less
Are we are not one with the Great
  Mother's heartbeat
the universal pulse
as she crashes on the shore or
  whispers in the wind

for we are bound together in the
  universal web of life
I feel I have always been a nurse
I know I will always be a nurse
forever in the moment, changing,
  transforming
striving for wholeness
timeless, spaceless.

(Gully 1998)

Journey to the soul

Reflective practice brings us closer to the self, to the 'I' of who we are within our nursing practice. It enables a metamorphosis, an awakening of the self and a finding of the sacred path of personal knowing and being, within the art and science of nursing practice. I share with you my journey to this beginning of knowing. I know that this is not the path all nurses choose or even want to take; though for some this may be the way they come to deepen their practice and of course their personal career satisfaction.

As I walked the length of the beach, my back garden, my mind wandered back to the years that had gone and I reflected in truly awesome wonder at what had shaped my life and living. I have spent years working with souls who faced life-threatening and challenging illness, and hours with those who prepared for their final transition: the last stage of their personal growth and development, death. I know that my life has been enriched by these encounters and the confidences I have been privileged to share. The treasure I hold in my heart of 'the other's soul journey' enables me to share some aspects of those ordinary, everyday experiences, in the hope that they will enrich other travellers on this life journey to open to the gifts that suffering, death and dying impart. Now is the time to give back to the profession I honour and love, and to share those stories with others.

Our lives and worldview are shaped, for the most part, by the values and beliefs of our culture, religion, family and life experiences. This worldview remains largely unchallenged until some experience or new learning comes our way to open our eyes. Of course for the change to come about in our worldview, we need to keep our hearts open and receptive. I say this because unless we are open to change, our lives remain the same and we are less enriched spiritually and personally.

I would like to share three unique stories with you as exemplars of how I weave contemplative reflection into my experiential nursing practice. The first story speaks of how childhood beliefs may shape the worldview of the adult: Mary's story. The second speaks of how the child who was not raised in a specific paradigm or belief system creates a personal reality of hope in the face of death: James's story. The third is of a wymyn whose life was shaped by rigid values and beliefs; whose hope was shattered through childhood abuse; and of how she reached peace and forgiveness in her dying: Dianne's story. This third narrative lays bare the human effect of how weaving two opposing paradigms may shape and mould a soul as it prepares for the final stage of life, death. The fear and guilt fade into insignificance as the awareness and practice of unconditional love and forgiveness open the soul to new possibilities. Mary's and James's stories lay the foundation for the story of Dianne which formed the framework for a case study; the telling is more time involving and explicit so bear with me.

Mary's story

"A story I heard as a child from my educators highlights how a worldview might be shaped and affect one's life view. This was told to our class as preparation for our first Holy Communion, with a view to impressing on us the importance of having a pure heart before taking the body of Christ. The fear engendered from this story stayed with me for years and in part guided my initial path in life.

Mary, a seven-year-old, had died. Her funeral was at the church that was attached to the local parish school; the entire school was at her Requiem Mass. The air was heavy with grief and loss, the parents overwhelmed at the loss of one so small and gentle. They had taken comfort in the knowledge that she had received the last rites of the church and her journey and entry into heaven were their only consolation. Here she would wait for them, pray for them and be their guardian angel. Tears abounded yet the hope of the resurrection, new life after death, sustained the faithful. During the service a triple knock was heard. It seemed to emanate from the small white coffin. No one moved and the service continued, each one thinking it was his or her imagination or maybe it was a natural phenomenon of some sort. A few minutes later the knock was heard again, this time louder and more insistent; the stirring and whisperings in the congregation were now audible. A silence descended in the church as the priest turned to face his flock. No one moved; the fear was palpable. The priest moved from the altar to the coffin and again the knock was heard. Quickly the lid was raised, for fear the child was to be buried alive. The body lay still in death; Mary's hands were clasped on her breast with her rosary entwined through her fingers. Her tongue protruded from her mouth, and on her tongue lay the communion host; her tongue was black. Shock and horror filled the souls of the faithful. Here was a child whose entry to heaven had been assured and now the deepest doubt filled the very core of the united congregation. The priest enlightened the faithful with the explanation that Mary had not confessed all her sins and had died in sin without forgiveness. So, we were told by our elders, 'If you die in sin, your soul is damned for eternity.' From then on, what kept some of us as children on the right path to salvation was fear of hell's fire and eternal damnation. Today, as an adult, care of the soul holds a different perspective for me. It has its foundation in love and respect for others, not fear and damnation.

Young minds are vulnerable and receptive; the memories of such stories have the capacity to paralyse an inquiring mind. There were many such stories told from a desire to keep us pure and on the right track in life. What sin, I asked myself in later years, could a seven-year-old child commit that had the potential to damn her soul to hell forever and destroy the hope of her loving parents?

It is hard to understand why people speak in this way. Although times have changed for the better, there are still souls who live with the scars of such teaching. When the time of death comes, this fear resurfaces and torment of the soul increases the pain and suffering of the deathing process. Many of those I have sat with during this journey have voiced their fear and spiritual anguish at having to face a wrathful God for the sins of their past. Their fear is that they can never be forgiven and they face eternal damnation.

For many years I lived the life of a semi-enclosed religious sister. This means I had very little to do with the outside world. I took this path at the age of fifteen for fear of losing my faith and of making the wrong choices in life, for fear of the loss of my own soul, but above all to do something with my life that would bring joy to my mother. Because of the nature of the work that was done by the Community of Sisters I was with, I would have occasion to sit with the dying during the wee small hours of the night. My own childhood fears would return: fear that the devil would appear in some gruesome form and snatch the soul of the dying person before my very eyes. I would pray till my heart ached and my fingers were numb from toiling my rosary beads. My life was fear. In those days we were not trained in the art of caring for the dying, rather to bear witness to the salvation of the Christian soul. And I questioned not! Would a loving God want this? This question did not come for many years. I soaked the essence of ritual into my very being, believing all that was told me. I was unaware of other ways of serving humankind that have the potential to open the doors of opportunity for others and myself to discover meaningful ways of being in the world.

The experience of illness brought me wisdom and clarity, such is the nature of this occurrence for some; the scales of ignorance and naïveté gradually fell from my soul. With an eye of longing I sought new knowledge and experiences. I had a thirst for truth, knowledge and understanding that led me to question my worldview and to grow spiritually. I discovered a new world, my path changed and old beliefs and values were transformed. My spiritual quest had begun, inviting my soul to delve deeper into the unknown and seemingly unknowable.

As I left my former life behind, taking with me the valuable experiences I had gained, I journeyed through life with greater intensity and purpose. I trained as a nurse, counsellor and healer, working with people who suffered life-threatening and challenging illnesses. I wanted to share my insights with those who feared the final stage of this journey, to open doors that would shed light and love on the soul's journey to health and wholeness even in death; and create sacred space to enable the process of self-transformation.

Nature has become my church, my strength and source of contemplative meditation. In silent contemplation I seek solitude to quieten the mind and soul and nourish the spiritual being I am. For such is our destiny to grow and develop as spiritual beings, to find the sacred space within, devoid of fear and full of unconditional love and forgiveness. Fear has the potential to paralyse and close the eyes of the soul to the innate human potential of love and growth. I bear witness to this in the moments I have shared with the dying."

Here now is the story of a young boy who suffered a life-threatening illness. This story serves to illustrate the antithesis of the narrow worldview from Mary's paradigm.

James's story

"James was 7 years old and had cancer. For reasons other than his illness alone, he remained in hospital for nearly a year. The nursing staff grew to love this little boy and did much to ease the pain and sadness in his young life. Following the failure of intensive treatment to rid his little body of the offending cells, James underwent a bone marrow transplant and was cared for in isolation. Isolation and loneliness were relieved by the constant presence of the nurses. Time passed and newly developed cells heralded a new beginning. This miracle was short lived, and James's body succumbed to yet another invasion. Time was running out and he had yet to be told of his impending death. Children are often intuitive and have a sense of the mysteries of life; they experience life without the judgements and fear of adults, as their life experiences have not shaped a negative perspective or life view.

Each day a nurse was assigned to James. For some nurses, caring for James was heart breaking and it was difficult for them to face this little boy with hope and optimism. I was to care for James this particular day. Together we chose to have some fun. James loved music; we played tunes he could move about to. There were a couple of songs at that time that were popular with the young people: 'I should be so lucky' and 'Do the locomotion with me'. Together we danced, swinging drip poles and all, masks and gowns to boot. Between infusions and care nothing could hold us back. It was hot, dancing with all the protective gear on!

Without warning, James asked, 'Am I going to die?' His eyes pleaded for an answer from the heart and for truth. I gently asked him, 'What do you think, James? What do you feel?' James replied that because he had been in his room for so long, he knew he was not getting better and that he thought he would die. For a moment I was stunned by the question. What should I tell him, and how much should I tell him? James sat on the bed and the tears in his eyes begged a response of truth. 'Where will I go?' he asked. 'What will it be like?' Questions asked by so many faced with death. This was a precious moment in the life of James, and I needed to gather all my strength to work at a deep soul level; to let go of my own emotions and be present in the moment with this child. My youngest child was not much older than James was.

Gathering coloured pens and bright paper we sat on the bed ready to create something. I had to believe that the right words would be gifted to me in this moment. I told him the story of *The Very Hungry Caterpillar* (Carle 1969), a story my children loved to hear. Taking the art materials we began to draw the pictures from the story; we cut out the images and laid them on the bed beside us. James looked with pride on the work he had done. A big black egg on a green leaf, the hatching of the caterpillar, the plant stalks that gave witness to the voracious appetite of the insect, the cocoon hanging precariously from a stalk and finally a beautiful butterfly, bright and shiny, stared back at us as we sat side by side on the hospital bed. 'Now what?' he asked. With paste and string we made a hanging mobile and hung it over the end of James's bed. Again we shared the story of the very hungry caterpillar, only this time it was James who was the egg, the caterpillar, the cocoon and finally the butterfly, which flew freely. We drew images of the process of living and dying from the mobile and the final metamorphosis. We shared the song:

Butterfly fair day is dead
Lift your wings and show your head
Spread your wings and fly away
For one sweet summer day.

James was quiet for a while, then asked if he would fly away and be beautiful. It is hard to hold back the tears when one so young shows such insight and pure faith in the face of death. Together we hugged as best we could for fear of disrupting the medical paraphernalia that James was attached to. James cried a little and was reassured to know that he would not be alone; we would be there to witness his amazing transformation with song and music, deep love and compassion.

I believe together James and I created sacred space in that isolation room, where the story momentarily transformed fear into hope, sadness into anticipation. Here the image of the chrysalis was seen as a state of inner self-reflection and contemplation, and what emerged was a metaphor for what we call dying and death. An awesome butterfly of colour and light and in flight understood the pain of self-transformation and metamorphosis.

Yes, we would miss James, but each time we saw a butterfly we would be reminded of him and send him a kiss. He would never be forgotten. James was special, as all children are. He did not have images of hell and fire to scare him; he had something more precious by far. He would be free to fly, to face his death without fear, and he would be surrounded with love. James died peacefully and we mourned his loss and marvelled at his courage and specialness. The gift James left us was one of unconditional love and trust."

The case study and its relation to theory

The two preceding stories are poles apart. One speaks of fear and the other tells of unconditional love, anticipation and hope in the face of inevitable death.

I offer you this next story, a case study, as an interweaving of the two previous ones. This is an exemplar of my nursing practice and reveals how my own life experiences have paved the way for this reflective narrative; this wymyn's story is presented as a journey, a search for inner healing from the pain and suffering of childhood, and personal transformation through attending to the work of the soul with loving compassion.

The essence of this case study is soulwork, a phenomenon rich in texture and pregnant with contextual meaning for inner healing and personal transformation. The narrative explores the theme of soulwork within the theory, science and practice of humanistic nursing. It is in essence located in the transpersonal caring relationship theory of Watson (1995), and the humanistic science of Patterson & Zderad (1988).

I took inspiration for the study from the work of such authors as John of the Cross (1570–81), Keegan (1994), Dossey *et al.* (1995) and Moore (1996). I believe these authors speak to the heart of any person who wishes to delve more deeply into the phenomenon of the soul and its essence.

> Nurses act as imaginative artists calling forth the actualities of a patient by being open to the unique possibilities in a situation . . .
>
> (Patterson & Zderad 1988)

Working with the soul of another in the context of nursing practice opens us as nurses to unique opportunities for our own spiritual development, for often we are privy to the inner soul expression of those in our care.

What differentiates this method of research from others is that I as the nurse respond with my being in the relationship with the other, a concept that does not fit with other methods of research. Of course there will always be important differences between myself and the other person, for this creates equality within the relationship (Patterson & Zderad 1988).

I believe that soulwork within the art of nursing has the potential to offer wisdom and insight to those with whom we walk the sacred path of personal inner healing. Soulwork empowers and assists people who experience a life-threatening/challenging illness in their quest for the meaning and purpose of their existence. I do not claim to know what happens to the person when working with the soul; what I do know is that change occurs and that together we move into a space that enables that change to occur.

The design is a retrospective single case study and sought to reveal the practice research findings. Case study offers a way of research that is, of its very nature, founded on the relationship between the lived experience, expression and understanding of individual experience in relation to another's (Hutchinson 1990; Yin 1994; Stake 1995). Case studies are important to nursing in that they emphasise and focus on the contemporary phenomenon within real-life situations (Yin 1994). Hutchinson (1990) suggests that the particulars of a case study be used to build theory for nursing practice and are a primary vehicle for emic inquiry.

The aim of the research was to create an understanding of the essence and meaning of soulwork within my practice of humanistic nursing. As nursing is both an art and a science, this work sits well in the qualitative methodology (Schultz & Kerr 1986). My intention was to reveal the spiritual complexities of soulwork within the art of nursing and in so doing to create a human face to the personal experience of pain, suffering and anguish within everyday nursing practice.

The methodology is steeped in hermeneutics, that is, the theory and practice of interpretation and understanding of different kinds of human experience (Odman 1988). The story is multilayered, providing a way of unravelling shared experiences and clarifying the complexities of care in my practice. This is not an analytical work; rather a synthesis and a weaving of the phenomenon of soulwork within the ethical boundaries of safe practice, theory and care. Humanistic case study illuminates human experience and real life problems, which are sometimes overlooked by other scientific approaches (Hutchinson 1990). Practice theory is my way of working with the other in the therapeutic relationship: humanistic research provided the conduit for the exploration and elucidation of this work.

Watson (1995) suggests that the practice theory is an imaginative grouping of knowledge, ideas and experience that are represented symbolically and seek to illuminate a given experience. I believe this to be how I work with others to create my own theory of soulwork. When I work with the soul of another, I know that my imagination stirs me to seek out new ways to open the other person to their own soulwork journey. These ways take the shape of ritual, music, meditation, human touch, active visualisation and the process of grounding and centring, and the use of art, poetry and reflective journaling, both for the therapeutic use of myself and to prepare the other for the healing process. I am aware that together we create sacred space. I do not direct, rather I work to facilitate an environment where the other person is enabled to articulate her/his own needs, for this is the nature of soulwork.

The people we meet on our life journey offer many gifts for our own personal growth and spiritual enlightenment; the research offered me precious spiritual insights and the gift of writing. I believe the experiences we are given in life are not serendipitous, they are given to us as an offering, providing us with the opportunity for deep spiritual enrichment. What is expected of us is that we keep an open heart, and we practise inner reflection and mindful contemplation. By this I mean the ability to create the time and space in daily life to connect with our inner world of personal spirituality. Spirituality demands practice. However, the benefits we receive enrich our living with deep peace and harmony and give purpose to the ordinary and sometimes wearisome tasks of daily existence. This is soulwork.

Soul, I believe, is the essence of our very being, the spirit that lies deep within each of us. What is asked of us is that our spiritual growth or soul manifestation is given time and space to grow. Nourishing the soul, as we do the body, creates the environment for our own innate potential to heal the hurts of the past and allow us to live in the present moment free of the effects of old wounds and the weight of personal baggage.

Soulwork offers us as nurses the opportunity to explore the meaning and purpose of our own existence and, when working with the other in nursing practice, to find the joy of empowerment of the other to seek their own meaning to their life experiences. Soulwork requires us to use our imagination, creativity and commitment. If we as nurses ignore the work of our own soul, is it possible to enter the journey of another who experiences illness and meet that person's needs efficaciously? Working with the soul is the foundation of my practice. The journey I shared with the other became my journey too. The writing of this research/soul journey was a spiritual gift, for it enabled me to articulate the very essence of my practice (Gully 1998).

The journal: a tool for reflective practice

Reflective practice is part of the way I work with others in my nursing practice. Journaling my reflective thinking is the way I make sense of the events and encounters; it is the process that enriches the therapeutic nursing relationship. Journaling is both a professional and personal way of making sense of everyday living. It may be called a journey to wholeness and well being. It is the process of journaling that is by far the most significant act in my practice, for it records the process of my evolving as a human being and connects me with the other in my nursing relationship; it is a journey from the 'I' to the 'we', the consciousness of the collective soul journey of each human being. The journey begins with the self, the awakening to the self, in relation to the spiritual path each of us is destined to follow. I hold the strong belief within my practice that I cannot walk the spiritual journey with another unless I have opened my self to my own (see Figure 11.1). For the case study research I kept a record of my thoughts, insights and shared experiences, careful to note when I was out of balance and mindful of boundaries and parallel processes. I explored the concept of mindfulness in depth, aware that this phenomenon prepared me for the gift of a richer understanding of the concepts of presence and being within the therapeutic relationship and the gift of understanding at a deep soul level. Soulwork is the creative and imaginative energy of the human spirit. I found the use of reflective practice and the keeping of a journal during this process to be invaluable.

In the writing of the retrospective case study I was mindful of the responsibility regarding the question of personal interpretation and integrity. As the keeper/guardian of this account, I honoured the invitation to share this with others within the bounds of an ethical process. Family members were included, as were significant others. They were invited to read the text at various intervals, and invited to make any changes they deemed necessary; sensitivity and compassion were paramount. There was the issue of self-disclosure, which precipitated personal self-reflection and constant evaluation; these issues were addressed through regular supervision.

Walking The Sacred Path

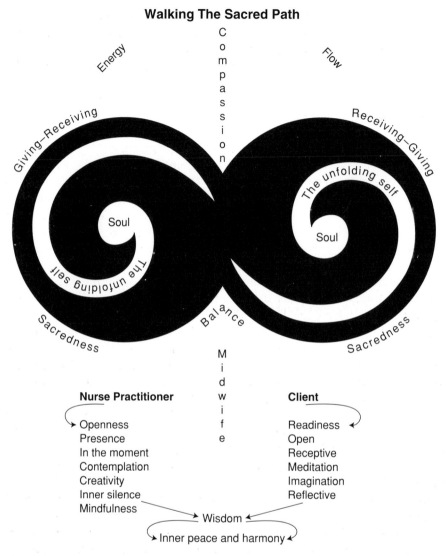

Figure 11.1   The innate healing process. From Gully 1998.

The narrative is multilayered and may be read as a text or as a personal journey where the images created become profoundly personal and intimate experiences.[1] The sacred path of spiritual growth knows no bounds; it calls each of us in ways that are recognisable and acceptable to our own lifestyle.

This is a story, a case study of an ordinary wymyn who faced her challenge extraordinarily well and had the courage and strength to turn her life around.

---

[1] In the original case study, the presence of photography, artwork and poetry are integral to the work for they sit as an aesthetic presence and bridge the gap between the spoken and unspoken words in the therapeutic relationship. They give the reader the opportunity to use personal and creative imagination to the understanding of this work.

Before her death she challenged me to write her story and take it to the nursing world. She wanted everyone to know the beauty of the journey of soulwork and the value of the nurse/client therapeutic relationship.

This is my interpretation of that experience, for how could it be otherwise?

Dianne's story

"It was a Sunday afternoon when I first heard from Dianne. She had heard of my private practice through a mutual friend and now requested my help in a time of personal crisis. At this time I was working as an oncology nurse and had a private practice as an independent nurse practitioner/counsellor. Some two years previous to this encounter, Dianne had had surgery for bowel cancer; she believed at the time that all evidence of the disease has been removed, that she had beaten it, and was well on the way to recovery. The six-monthly check-up indicated liver metastasis and Dianne was told her cancer had returned; she was in a state of shock and disbelief at the news of her condition. How was it possible for her to be in good health and symptom free and yet still have the cancer? She could not make sense of this new revelation.

Following our first session, Dianne and I contracted to work together for the long haul. As it happened this took around 18 months. As the months unfolded, Dianne shared her life's story with me. It became evident that her way of being in the world had been in part shaped by her childhood experience of incest and the unhealthy silence that haunted her growing up.

Dianne's challenge was to face her shadow self, her demons of the past, and attend to the work of her soul. Initially Dianne set out to beat the cancer. As time went on she realised that this was not to be. Cancer was her experience, her gift and eventually her legacy to the world within the context of the caring nursing relationship.

Deeply embedded within Dianne was intense anger, and a need to control situations in her life. This worked against her and set her up for relationship failures both within and around her family. Dianne knew in her soul that inner healing was the path she needed to take; this knowledge was emancipatory. Our work together opened the way for her to explore the patterns in her life that were no longer useful and attend to the work of her soul, to enable her to find peace and harmony and restore family relationships.

Dianne was a fighter, and her body and verbal language were evidence of this. She committed herself with courage and determination to changing her life around, through the phenomenon of working with her soul. Our work together was a turning point in time; a time when we shared our humanity, enabling an inward journey to a deep spiritual awakening for both of us. Over the months of our working together at soul level, Dianne found the gentle side of herself; her body language softened and she learned to love and trust those close to her."

How did this transformation happen, and what do I mean by working with the soul within the context of nursing practice? I would like to offer you

my insight into what I understand to be the work of the soul in the caring relationship. Second I will demonstrate through Dianne's story how the process
came about.

When we look at the phenomenon of working with the soul, it invites
the question of how this fits within the context of nursing practice. There is
sacredness about this work. As such, issues such as the ethic of care, the protection of personal and client boundaries, and congruence and trust require
integrity and constant personal reflection on the part of the nurse practitioner.
As a nurse I cannot separate myself from my nursing practice for my deep
connection with my practice is rooted within the work of the soul.

Thomas Moore (1996) tells us that to define soulwork or soul is an
intellectual exercise. Soul is not a thing, rather a quality, or a dimension of
experiencing life and ourselves. Soul has to do with depth, heart and personal
substance. Soul is the essence of who we are in relation to human existence.
Soulwork explores creativity and imagination in the work of finding who we
are in the world, the meaning and purpose of our human existence. I believe
that soulwork is life longing for itself, searching for meaning to life's experiences and mysteries (John of the Cross 1570–81) Having experienced this
personally within the context of my own life, I wanted to share this with
Dianne, that she would find her own meaning of her experiences. In the telling
of her story, the vision is inevitably my own.

Soulwork opens to us the innate healing potential and from that flows a
connectedness with the collective world consciousness and world healing.
Soulwork is our own deep inner wisdom, transforming existential experiences
into a meaningful and purposeful way of being in the world.

Dianne plunged into the depths of her soulwork with fear and trepidation,
afraid of the emotion that had been buried for so long, afraid of what she
would find. It was for her a Pandora's box. My part was to be there for her. We
had made a covenant to work together for the 'long haul'. Neither of us knew
how this would look, and the landscape was unclear as we steered into the
unknown. For my part I sought constant supervision from a wymyn who
shared a similar worldview and understood the depth of the work Dianne and
I had undertaken. There were times when I felt exhausted with the demands
of the work and sought refuge through contemplation and reflection in quiet
retreat. I had never worked with someone who held so much anger and
had hurt for so long. For any therapeutic relationship to unfold, the foundation blocks of mutual trust, voluntary openness and willingness for personal
change and transformation are required. Dianne shared her experiences and
together we sought ways of working with them, for the essence of working
with the soul is about what can be done with the experiences, not what can
be done about them (Gully 1998).

The philosophy of my nursing practice is founded on the practice of contemplation, awareness and attention to the work of my own creative soul. In my
work with Dianne I moved beyond myself as an individual and endeavoured
to keep my own ego in abeyance, to ensure that Dianne's needs were met
within the ethical bounds of safe practice. This process is central to my practice

of working with the soul for it is through my own transpersonal self-healing and awareness that I as the nurse am able to meet another person in soul time and sacred space. I believe I cannot walk the path with another unless I have walked the path myself. I have included a model and explanation of what I believe is the foundation for the exploration of the sacred path (Figure 11.1).

Exploring the sacred path

The symbols of the two *koru* (spirals) represent the journey of the two soul travellers in soul time and space. The symbolic image of the *koru* represents reciprocity, inner reflection and silence. The ongoing weaving motion of the *koru* draws attention to the journey's inner and outer movement. It speaks to the reader of the endlessness of the soul journey and reveals the potential of the soul's unfolding self. The destination is unimportant; the journey in itself holds the unfolding mystery of the soul's awakening.

What is asked of each person in the process of unfolding the self is a readiness, an opening and receptivity in walking the sacred path. Meditation is the channel through which the soul prepares itself for inner silence and contemplation (Watson 1995). Meditation is the preparation of the soul for the seed from which the gift of mindfulness grows. Mindfulness is the art of being fully alive and of having an awareness of every precious aspect of life (Thich 1987).

The entwined *koru* speak of the masculine and feminine energies of the soul and the continuous movement to achieve unity and balance within the soul's centre. When balance between the energies is found, the soul opens to wisdom and a sense of inner peace and harmony is experienced.

Walking the sacred path opens the soul to the innate healing potential and a deep connection and harmony with all life and world soul. The soul journey enables the individual to develop and enrich the personal power in their lives. Personal power is no more than an awareness and use of one's own personal, creative and imaginative gifts and abilities. Soul journeying is a sacred art and restores a sense of the spiritual dimension in life.

This model of walking the sacred path has served me well on my own spiritual journey. It is with humility that I offer it to others who feel they might be drawn to caring for their own soul and that of those who experience a life-threatening/challenging illness (Gully 1998).

Our relationship began with Dianne's narrative, and from her story we explored the patterns that had flowed through her life. One of these patterns was as we have already mentioned: that of how her anger had tainted her relationships. This anger pushed away those she loved the most. Why had this happened? Following a lengthy process Dianne realised she had always felt alone and unworthy, and held the secret of incest in her soul. From the age of 4 years she had known that her mother was aware of it and had done nothing to keep her safe. Dianne felt dirty and harboured a deep self-loathing. How could anybody love her or even want her? Her self-love, self-worth and personal integrity were, to say the least, marginalised. She left school in her early teens and sought comfort in many transient relationships. She feared for the safety of her younger sister and did all she could to protect her. Hear her voice as she speaks to us of how she felt:

Who am I
Who am I
I feel like nothing
don't know who I am
who the real me is.
I wear different hats
mother
grandmother
bus operator
friend
ex wife and lover, partner
child
I work, love, laugh, cry,
dance, sing, drive,
read, cook, clean, wash, iron,
sew, shop, garden,
talk, write, listen to music,
watch telly, meditate, bath,
    shower,
exercise, walk, run.
But who is the real me?
Who am I?
I feel like a robot
except I feel I have feelings.
Ever since I was a child I've been
Fucked Over

Mentally, physically
I've lost myself somewhere
In the anger
sadness
hurt
bewilderment
in the growing up too soon
tears
food
abuse
I feel a hole
a void
a gaping wound
deep inside of me.
'I' am somewhere deep inside this
I need to know who the real 'me' is
who I really am
what I really am.
I know I am strong also I'm very
    vulnerable
Frightened what if I find nothing
a nobody
maybe I don't exist
never did never will
am I a figment of the imagination?
I feel cold

(Dianne Frances 1993)

The words stand alone and need no interpretation for they come from the depth of her very being.

Through processes such as meditation, visualisation, and therapeutic and healing touch and massage, Dianne opened the gate to her consuming anger and pent-up emotions. She was vulnerable, yet resolute in her journey to the unfolding self. She was now able to verbalise her emotions, her hatred and sense of injustice that had been her burden from childhood.

Never the time
Frustration, waiting, holding on
    to it all
Is the story of my life.
Bury it, put it away, don't show it now.
Anger is not allowed

Never the right time
Not appropriate
Can't connect and touch base
Miss by moments
Not fair
Life's not fair never has been

(Dianne Frances 1993)

She spoke of the anger as a 'chewing in her gut'. Now she could look at the anger that had almost consumed her and deal with it; search her soul about what to do with it. Dianne wanted to find who she was. She understood her dis ease to be a metaphor; a way to perceive her inner and outer world and create meaning and synthesis of her life experiences. She understood that what had happened in her body through the cancer 'chewing at her gut', was a metaphor for what was happening in her soul through her life experiences (Walzlawick 1978 cited in Breslin 1996).

She had learned to set up a sacred space in her own home. She described this as a quiet place for herself, surrounding it with objects and rituals that were important to her alone. This space was used for visualisation and the practice of meditation and quiet reflection. Dianne practised these rituals for months. However hard she tried, too hard sometimes, she could not find inner peace; such is the all-consuming power of unresolved anger.

One evening, following a massage, Dianne shared with me what had happened for her during this process. The room was softly lit with candlelight, the therapeutic aroma of lavender filled the air and the haunting sound of Terry Oldfield's[2] music gently vibrated around us. Dianne said she saw her deceased father; she gazed into his eyes and he into hers for what seemed like an eternity; she commented that the vision was wordless. Dianne said that following this time with her father, she was filled with a peaceful sense of unconditional love and forgiveness for her parents. This differed markedly from other sessions, where she had felt hatred and relentless unforgiving for her father. This was a moment of transformation. Following each process Dianne would be invited to draw or write what she experienced. Her poetry is a legacy to her feeling and emotions.

Gateway

Visualisation of myself	Everything it took to bring me here
Standing before a gateway	Observe it all
My entire life behind me and below	Bless it all
I pause and review the past	By letting go of the past
The learning and the joys	I reclaim my power
The victories and the sorrows	Step through the gateway now.

(Dianne Frances 1994)

Following the night when she opened herself to her own soul's journey, when she quieted her mind and was in the moment, the experience of her daily ritual changed. Dianne gave up forcing herself to move in her soul's journey, and the peace she had so longed for emanated from within. It is not what we do in the journey of the unfolding self, rather a letting go and a stilling of the mind, that transforms our way of being in the world.

---

2 Terry Oldfield 'Out of the Depths' (De Profundis), New World Company (1993).

Dianne had been born and raised as Catholic but she felt the Catholic community had not been there for her in her childhood. She felt her soul was damned. Through each and every process we shared in the therapeutic relationship, Dianne found more and more of her soul – beautiful and vibrant. She reflected on her life and experiences and found meaning to her existence and her cancer. She explored her own uniqueness and creativity, using her imagination to spark the flame of life in each living moment.

There were times we spent at the beach or the rocks and felt the spray of the ocean on our faces. Dianne would disclose more of her pain and lost love, the wounding of her sons and daughter and wonder how she might find the way to restoring the love and trust that had been lost over the years. Through the birth of her first granddaughter the first steps to reconciliation were made. Dianne talked of her daughter who had died at 2 years of age and for whom she had not grieved. She felt that her daughter had come back as her grandchild and she was able to love her and hold her as she had never done for her first child. She grieved for her loss and rejoiced in her gain. Dianne had a peace about her now, and knew how to access that peace in times of trouble and stress. This was the miracle of mindfulness and being present in the moment. When she was told there was no further medical treatment available to her, she accepted this with equanimity of soul and mind and deep peace. She resolved to die with peace and dignity. Having rekindled family relationships and assured them of her unconditional love, she prepared for her death. They were with her in her dying, supportive and loving. The last words Dianne spoke to me were: 'I want to go with dignity. I feel peaceful inside. Different things are important now' (Gully 1998).

The art of nursing enabled the bridging of the gap between Dianne's disease and the experience of her illness. Dianne's pain taps into the collective pain of all humankind for we are bound together in the universal web of life; this phenomenon is what I call world soul for it connects us to nature and the land. What happens in the human body through dis ease may be seen as a metaphor for what is taking place in the land. The rivers, streams and seas of the world are clogged with pollution and as a consequence the Earth and humankind suffer. These are nursing issues, for how are we able to find health and wholeness in a world that has been ravaged and uncared for by humankind?

As we are called to care for ourselves through soulwork, so too are we called to care for the soul of the world through caring communities and care of Mother Earth. World soul or soul of the world is a way of referring to the collective human connection we have to nature and the land, in which we live and have our being. There is a delicate balance that holds humanity and our ecology within the web of life, for we are so closely connected and inter-dependent. This is a deep wordless connection that is beyond theory or physical scientific explication. The belief that this deep connection between ourselves and the natural world holds the potential for the unfolding of the intangible spiritual self, as it weaves through our inner and outer world, enables us to experience a harmony within our soul and ecology. It may be that the manifestations of the ills of modern society are related to our loss of connection with nature, thus creating an imbalance in our lives and a disconnection from our soul wisdom and world soul. Maybe we have lost sense of the sacred in our own lives. The caring relationship through soulwork inspires the innate human potential of self-healing. It offers us insight of a deep spiritual significance and may in part restore the imbalance in our communities and in our world. In a small way this exemplar offers a beacon of hope to those of us who share the passion for humanistic nursing.

Dianne wanted her story known to the nursing community to demonstrate how the therapeutic relationship within the context of nursing practice met her need for personal transformation and self-healing. We all have the capacity for self-healing. Sometimes we just need encouragement and caring, compassionate support. Through the experience of illness Dianne found the meaning and purpose of her existence; she discovered herself to be worthy of loving and being loved. Dianne accepted the challenge her illness offered her; to go within herself and walk the sacred path of inner knowing and spiritual growth. She honoured the work of her soul, and having achieved health and wholeness through her illness experience she died peacefully surrounded by her immediate family.

Dianne left an inspiring legacy to her family, to those who shared her journey and to the nursing profession. I honour her for her courage and trust, and for the gift she gave me of taking her story to the nursing world. It is with humility and gratitude that I have shared this story with you.

Linking the stories

I have used three stories from my life experience to demonstrate how we are shaped by our worldview, for this may limit us as we journey through life. The ritual of contemplative reflection on those sacred experiences in my practice has given me the opportunity to make sense of difficult and painful moments, to see the bigger picture, to change my worldview. I know that this is not the path all nurses choose or even want to take; for some this will be the way they come to deepen their practice and of course their personal career satisfaction. For myself, contemplative reflection is my *raison d'être*.

As much as this narrative is Dianne's story, it is inevitably mine in that it expresses my way of being, which has been informed and shaped by her story. I am who I am. I too was raised a Catholic along with my six sisters and four brothers. Religion was an integral part of our lives. Catholicism brought with it fear and guilt in the 1940s and 1950s: fear of sin and guilt. Anyone educated in the faith at this time will well identify with this comment. Loss of the faith and fear of losing one's soul was terrifying and had the power to paralyse creative and imaginative living. For many souls today, this way of being still haunts their life. I have heard the pain and suffering of many souls, just like Dianne, as they prepared for death, and I have had the privilege to share their opening to transformation and peace and to their aspiration to experience unconditional love and forgiveness through the journey to their soul. Walking the sacred path has the potential to lead us to our own inner wisdom and open doors of opportunity to inner peace and harmony.

The stories of Mary, James and Dianne will stay forever in my heart and guide me in the preparation for my own inevitable moment of final transition, death. These souls have inspired my living and being and made clear for me the way I want to be in the here and now. They have made me the person I am today, for these stories have shaped my thinking and inspired my nursing practice.

Full Circle

Often the end is the beginning
and the beginning is the end
as life unfolds on itself
one season moves into another in
   mysterious silence
I find myself in silent space
to give myself the gift of solitude
to be at one with the beat of the
   universe
heart to heart, beat for beat
shall I set myself a goal today or
   shall I just be
enjoying my being, at one with
   myself
in harmony and peace with the
   universe
beat for beat
rhythm beating harmony
pulsating through my veins
tireless movement

today I shall be
enjoying the taste
the luxury of being
its fruitfulness, bounty,
   loving
caring and joy
filling the vessel within
my soul overflowing
ready to pour again
sharing giving receiving
being
the rhythm of life
of birth and death
of loving and grieving
of being, compassion
life has come full circle
one season moves into another
in mysterious silence
often the end is the beginning
and the beginning is the end.

(Eleanor Gully 1997)

Life is a striving for the human capacity of living, loving and sharing compassion; such is my belief in the possibility that is gifted to us through working with the soul and the process of reflective nursing practice. The experiences I have shared from my practice have given me my deeper thirsting after life.

References

Breslin, E. (1996) Metaphor as aesthetic method for nursing practice. *Issues in Mental Health Nursing*, **17**: 507–16.

Carle, E. (1969) *The Very Hungry Caterpillar*. Hamish Hamilton, London.

Dossey, B., Keegan, L., Guzzetta, C. and Kolmeier, L. (1995) *Holistic Nursing: A Handbook for Practice*, 2nd edn. Aspen Publishers, Gaithersburg, MD.

Gibran, K. (1973) *The Prophet*. Heinemann, London.

Gully, E. (1998) A retrospective case of one wymyn's experience of a life threatening/challenging illness: Theme Soul work. Victoria University, New Zealand. Unpublished thesis.

Hutchinson, S. (1990) A case study approach. *Advancing Nursing Science through Research*, **2**: 177–213.

John of the Cross (1570–81) *The Ascent of Mount Carmel – The Dark Night*. In *The Collected Works of St John of the Cross* (Kavanaugh, K. & Rodriguez, O., transl. from the Spanish text *Biblioteca de Autores Espanoles* (1853). ICN Publications, Institute of Carmelite Studies, Washington, DC.

Keegan, L. (1994) *The Nurse as Healer*. Delmar Publishers, New York.

Moore, T. (1996) *The Re-enchantment of Everyday Life*. Hodder & Stoughton, London.

Odman, P. (1988) Hermeneutics. In *Paths to Knowledge. Educational Research, Methodology, and Measurement: An International Handbook* (Keeves, J.P., ed.). Pergamon, Oxford.

Patterson, J. and Zderad, L. (1988) *Humanistic Nursing*, 2nd edn. National League for Nursing, New York.

Schultz, P. and Kerr, B. (1986) Comparative case study as a strategy for nursing research. In *Nursing Research Methodology* (Chinn, P.L., ed.). Rockville, Aspen.

Stake, R. (1995) *The Art of Case Study Research*. Sage, Beverley Hills, CA.

Thich, N. (1987) *The Miracle of Mindfulness. A Manual on Meditation* (Mobi Ho, transl. from the Vietnamese text, *Phep la cua su tinh thuc*, 1974. Beacon Press, Boston.

Watson, J. (1995) Nursing's caring–healing paradigm as an exemplar for alternative medicine? *Alternative Therapies*, **1**(3): 64–9.

Yin, R. (1994) *Case Study Research: Design and Methods*, 2nd edn. Applied Social Science Research Methods Series, Vol. 5. Sage, Beverley Hills, CA.

Chapter 12

Constructing the Reflexive Narrative

Lou Jarrett and Christopher Johns

In this chapter we offer Lou's narrative as an exemplar of constructing and presenting the reflexive narrative. Lou is currently using guided reflection as a process of self-inquiry and transformation towards realising desirable practice as a lived reality. She works with people experiencing spasticity. Chris is her research supervisor.

We pose two related questions. First, how can transformation be adequately recognised? Second, how can transformation be adequately presented? In brief, our answer to the first question is to either construct or adopt a valid framework to mark the transformation (of realising desirable practice). My answer to the second question is to construct a reflexive narrative.

The essence of transformation is captured by Blackwolf and Gina Jones (1996):

> To design your future, visualize where you want to be, and then build the bridge from your present, to that place. Your vision becomes your destiny, and your bridge becomes your path. Assure your bridge is strong with a well-defined plan.
>
> Transcend and flow with time, yet be present with the moment. Like all the winged, in order to transcend, we, too, must be in movement. We must vibrate. Truth after truth reveals itself at each fluttering of our spiritual wings. Like the gradual shading of blue to green, we become, we live the transformations. It is as though we are in a cocoon within a cocoon, within a cocoon. The more truths we experience, the more we are set free in colorful flight. Always in movement, the different levels of consciousness we experience lead us to the next level. This is how we come to soar! (p. 54, cited by Johns & Freshwater 1998, pp. ix–x)

Clearly, a narrative must start at the beginning, although the beginning is always a certain moment in time; a moment of autobiographical history. The narrative can be visualised as *the bridge* between that moment and *that place*, a future that may be envisaged but is as yet unknown.

To reach that place requires *a vision* of that place even though the vision might change en route as we journey. As such, the narrative may commence with a rationale for holding a certain vision. In Johns' recent work *Being Mindful, Easing Suffering* (Johns 2004b), the preface to the narrative stated the author's vision in working as a nurse and complementary therapist within a hospice setting, namely: 'easing suffering and nurturing the growth of the other through the health–illness experience'. Such words establish the plot, yet what these words mean in practice is essentially a mystery to be revealed. Immediately a number of questions demand answers. What is the nature of suffering? How can it best be eased? Are we able to ease suffering? These are questions that focus our self-inquiry.

For practitioners who struggle to articulate a vision of desirable practice, answering these questions must be the primary task. Unless we know what it is we are trying to achieve, how can we work towards achieving it?

Here we are going to suspend the issue of vision in the air to continue unwrapping Blackwolf and Gina's words. What can we make of the words, 'Assure your bridge is strong with a well-defined plan'? Simply that constructing a narrative requires the utmost commitment and discipline. By commitment we mean that the practitioner's practice matters to him or her. Why else would he or she want to pay attention to it? Practitioners must value what they do and be committed to the transformative endeavour. It is not simply doing a one-semester course where one might scratch the surface of reflection. Being a reflective practitioner is about being mindful, a constant paying attention to self within the unfolding moment along the journey: *'Transcend and flow with time, yet be present with the moment.'*

> Each footstep isn't just a means to an end but a unique event in itself. The leaf has jagged edges. The rock looks loose.
>
> (Pirsig 1974, p. 208)

It is living a narrative and that it is why writing a narrative is so difficult – capturing this exquisite journey of being and becoming in all its complexity and indeterminateness. But we can try. We can write our stories using metaphors, analogy, poems: forms of expression that enable both the writer and the reader to access the subtlety and depth of lived experience transforming over time. So the journey needs to be carefully planned and each step itself reflected on. The main kit is the reflective journal and a guide to reflect with regularly; a guide who knows the different ways yet doesn't impose a particular way.

To follow well-worn steps may feel safe but the risk is that it is accepted on face value like most research methodologies. The journey must itself be a path of discovery: *'Truth after truth reveals itself at each fluttering of our spiritual wings.'* These truths are moments of insight and realisation. Transformation is the process, not the outcome. Indeed there is no outcome, simply the plot that gives the journey meaning – to realise the vision.

The idea of the reflective journey being spiritual acknowledges that transformation is always to higher forms of consciousness involving the whole being of the person. Such acknowledgement moves reflection steeply away from mere cognitive or intellectual activity into meaning about existence. Perhaps to those of you who like us work with people who are suffering, the spiritual aspect of work is more obvious; yet such work is itself spiritual. It can be nothing less. Yet in a technologically driven world, many people may squirm and react against the idea of reflection as spiritual. Why do they contain themselves and close down this possibility? As we come to know and realise ourselves, we are liberated in colourful flight and can soar!

> Like the gradual shading of blue to green, we become, we live the *transformations*. It is though we are in a cocoon within a cocoon, within a cocoon.

These words capture the reflexive effort. Nothing is ever static along the reflective journey. Like water running continuously on limestone, it will make an impression. It is an important realisation that transforming self may take time, yet always needs discipline, patience and courage.

To return to the question, how can the reflexive or transformative journey be adequately marked? The practitioner has a choice whether to utilise existing *valid* interpretive frameworks or to construct his or her own. By valid, we mean it has to reflect the nature of desirable practice. The practitioner must critique the appropriateness of the proposed framework for its 'validity'. The use of valid frameworks grounds the practitioner's experiences within the wider body of knowledge, and in doing so contributes to the narrative's validity as a whole (see Johns 2002 for exploration of validity in guided reflection research).

In the following narrative Lou uses the 'being available' template (Box 12.1) to mark her development towards realising desirable practice. She chose this framework simply because it offered a reasonable representation of the holistic practice she endeavoured to realise in her everyday practice – being available to the person in order to help the person find meaning in their (health–illness) experience, to make best decisions, and to assist the person to take appropriate action to meet their health needs.

Frameworks can be less embracing, to focus on a particular quality of desirable and effective practice, for example using frameworks for empowerment of which a number have been constructed (Kieffer 1984; Belenky *et al.* 1986; Roberts 2000). Given nursing's interprofessional history it is perhaps

Box 12.1   The Being Available template (adapted from Johns 2004a)

The core therapeutic of nursing practice is the practitioner's being available to the other (patient/family) in order to guide them to find meaning in their health–illness experience so as to make best decisions about their health/lives, and to appropriately assist them to meet their health needs.

The ability of the practitioner to be available is determined by the extent the practitioner:

- has a strong valid vision of practice (the more the practitioner has a focused intent, the more likely it will be realised)
- is concerned for the other (the more concerned the practitioner, then the more attention given to the patient)
- appreciates the life pattern of the patient (the practitioner can only nurse what he or she knows about the patient's life)
- can make expert clinical decisions, respond with skilful action and reflect on the efficacy of action
- knows and manages self within relationship with equanimity
- can create and sustain a practice environment where being available is possible.

inevitable that empowerment will always be a key theme for nurses striving to realise their desirable practice in a culture that has traditionally dis-empowered them. A framework for being assertive has been constructed from analysing patterns of communication evident within experiences shared by practitioners within clinical supervision (Johns 2004a). Although Lou does not overtly use these frameworks in her exemplar, the text shouts out her empowerment quest.

Lou's narrative

In the following text, we present Lou's draft narrative over two guided reflection sessions and journal entries. The text is not a perfect exemplar because it is work in progress, yet it highlights a number of key points.

Janice, session 18: 15 October 2002

"I had known Janice and her husband for over four years. During this time she had used an implanted intrathecal baclofen (ITB) pump as part of her spasticity management. However, her symptoms were becoming more severe as her underlying disease process of multiple sclerosis progressed. Pressure sores on her sacrum and both heels were caused and exacerbated by difficulty in positioning her due to her level of spasticity, spasm and contracture. The ITB was no longer effective in reducing her spasticity and spasms, and she described being in constant agony with a deep gnawing pain, which was intensified every time she was touched or moved by her carers. This was negatively impacting on her mood, making her short tempered and irritable, and was placing a lot of tension on her close family relationships. In addition Janice was finding it harder to express her needs and was relying more and more on her husband to do this for her. The option of intrathecal phenol (IP) (see Box 12.2) and its associated potential side effects had been discussed on several occasions, and both Janice and her husband now decided it was time to see if it could be effective. In my journal I wrote:

> "They would need to come into hospital for a short admission. They both seemed anxious about this, but it is usual for people to be apprehensive about coming into hospital and I have noticed that I can try and ease the admission by informing the ward nurses about certain aspects of their care."

There is perhaps nothing out of the ordinary with this passage but through guided reflection I started to pay attention to how I use words and what impact this has on my practice and the way I perceive the individuals I work with. For instance, I write about the admission as if they are both coming into hospital, not just Janice. Is this significant in how I respect the husband's knowledge of Janice's care? Christopher Johns (CJ) asked why I wrote that people are *usually* apprehensive. Do I just assume that coming into hospital

Box 12.2   Technical data for intrathecal baclofen therapy and intrathecal phenol

---

Intrathecal baclofen therapy (ITB)

Baclofen is a GABA receptor agonist. Concentrations of GABA receptors are located at L2/3 in the spinal cord. Long-term management can be achieved with the use of an implanted pump system, which can deliver the drug directly to this site.

Issues

- Reduces spasticity, spasms and associated pain. Can help to improve function.
- Increases the effect and minimises side effects associated with oral baclofen.
- Requires a pump implant (approx. 2-week admission) which needs replacing every 5–7 years due to battery depletion.
- Needs regular outpatient visits to refill pump reservoir, on average every 2–3 months. Titration of dose to therapeutic level can take time, sometimes months.
- Allows flexible dosing over time. A pump can be programmed using telemetry to deliver different prescriptions over a 24-hour period.
- Side effects can include increase in weakness, drowsiness and difficulty breathing.
- Someone needs to be responsible for alerting hospital staff if problems develop with spasticity management and/or implanted system.

Further details can be found in Jarrett *et al.* 2001.

Intrathecal phenol

Phenol is a neurolytic chemical which when injected can stop the action of both motor and sensory nerves. This can be injected into the intrathecal space to target the muscles affected by the spasticity, i.e. hip and knee flexor, extensor or adductor muscles.

Issues

- Reduces spasticity, spasms and pain. Can improve comfort and ease of care.
- Requires expert injection.
- Can negatively affect bladder, bowel and sexual function; effective management strategies need to be instigated prior to injection.
- Can reduce lower limb sensation, therefore requires good skin care management.
- Initial 1-week hospital admission but then subsequent injections can be done as outpatient.

Further details can be found in Jarrett *et al.* 2002.

---

raises anxiety, or is something else happening here that is more specific? What did I mean by easing the admission? At this stage I couldn't really answer these questions, but it raised an awareness of part of my practice that I perhaps took for granted but could now start to question.

I discussed with Janice's husband the type of pressure-relieving mattress she would require and her husband pointed out other management techniques that had been refined by them with the community team; he was keen that these were not disrupted. One key issue was her bowel management: she requires enemas on Mondays, Wednesdays and Fridays to maintain her continence. This regime had been used over the past eight months and incontinence was now rare. It was clear that the husband could cope with all his wife's other needs but did find it difficult to manage faecal leakage. I assured him that I would pass this on to the ward team and we would endeavour to maintain the routine that was now working.

CJ questioned me. How could I be sure? Was I going to be there to monitor her care? How was I going to 'assure him'? Did I mean reassure, could I really do this, or was it a glib statement to say something in the short term to make them more confident about the admission? These questions resonated with how I try to practise. I do aim to make people feel less anxious and confident about coming into hospital, but am I doing this in the most effective way to maintain trust within our working relationship or am I giving them false hope by making promises I cannot keep? By giving glib reassurance for parts of her care that would be difficult for me to influence, am I not in danger of jeopardising my collaborative working relationship with this couple and of raising my own anxiety if their needs were not met?

I advised the nurses of a need for a mattress prior to the admission. Although a low-grade pressure-relieving mattress was available on admission, it was clear that Janice would need one of a higher standard and this took over 24 hours to arrive from stock. I was irritated that it was going to take 24 hours to meet this need despite prior planning. Further, throughout the admission, I constantly had to remind the nurses about her bowel management and how important it was to maintain it. This was despite describing the process that Janice, her husband and the community team had gone through, plus the management strategy being clearly written in the community care plan that accompanied her.

Was I taking a parental role? CJ thought so in response to managing my anxiety (framing this within a transactional analysis model). Rather than my negotiating with the family what I hoped the nurses would do, why had I not included the nurses in the discussion so that they could verify what they could do? How could I influence care on the ward? A potential solution could be to jointly assess the individual and plan care with the ward nurse admitting the person, so that we could all share knowledge and identify and solve potential difficulties early in the admission.

Janice's husband was also concerned that we would keep her in bed for long periods. He stated that she sat up for about 3–4 hours a day as it maintained her morale and made her cognitive impairment less evident. The ward and spasticity team agreed that outside the trials of treatment she should get up as normal. However, this seemed difficult to achieve. Her suprapubic catheter then started to block. The doctor changed it once, but the problem persisted. I asked the nurses if they had asked Janice's husband if this was a common feature. They had not, and when I spoke to him he said, 'Oh yes, it normally happens especially if she is lying in bed. It drains better when she is up.' The ward nurses wanted to nurse her in bed because of the catheter blocking, despite my feeding back what the husband had said and that the doctor was quite happy for Janice to get up.

Why was there so much resistance to follow what happened at home and to maintain Janice's individual routine? Why the reticence about communicating with her husband about what happens at home? Did they see her as ill rather than as having symptoms that we needed to find the best way to manage? True, some of the intrathecal treatments have risks of making someone unstable and that is why they have to be an inpatient, but this is not significant enough to abandon all other effective management techniques, which have taken targeted effort and time to perfect. Is my understanding of complex disability at odds with what the ward nurses believe? Is it a case of differing priorities? I decided to try to explore my understanding of the meaning of chronic illness.

- Disease is a condition of the body that causes symptoms that may or may not require treatment.
- Illness is when the disease process hits a crisis and requires medical, nursing and/or therapy intervention to sustain life.
- Chronic illness is a life-long disease process that can change over time and may need a series of adaptations or treatments to cope with and manage new or existing symptoms.
- Wellness is a successful management of symptoms to enable the individual to fulfil a chosen lifestyle or ease their approach to death and dying.

From this understanding it appears that my definition of illness is very narrow. I believe individuals with chronic illness can be in hospital but not be ill, instead requiring input to improve management of their symptoms (Harrison 1993). However, for nurses based on acute wards, there may be a belief that people are only admitted to hospital because they are ill, reaching an acute crisis, which will necessitate a full review of their care. I acknowledge that during the intrathecal treatments they may become ill and require expert intervention to ease them safely through, but this is when acute nursing expertise would prevail, not necessarily for all their care needs. From my perspective their 'illness' is short lived at different stages whilst in hospital. At other times we should try as far as possible to maintain their normal routine, listening to them and their carers, who are experts in their care, for directions.

   This could explain the tension between the ward nurses and myself that was further exacerbated by their apparent lack of concern to find out what happens at home. Are resources so restricted that nurses can only practise in a limited way, not enabling them to respond to the specific individual needs of people? Can nurses only react to hospital situations rather than plan and be proactive in finding out how individuals manage at home and how this can occur in hospital? What is my role: can I be more proactive at sharing what I know about patients prior to the day they are admitted so as to ease the transition in and out of hospital? Interestingly, one issue was relatively easy to solve. The ward sisters informed me that they were unable to order a high pressure-relieving mattress without the 'Waterlow score' (Waterlow 1985), hence the delay in ordering the correct mattress until the person had been assessed. Ironically I was already recording the Waterlow score in outpatients but not sharing it. Simply giving this to the ward nurses prior to admission is now speeding up the process of obtaining the correct mattresses."

This incident raised more questions and discrepancies between my desired and actual practice, but through the next incident we can see how these themes permeated and affected a subsequent admission.

Ann

"Ann has had an ITB pump implanted for 5 years. Recently in clinic the battery was shown to be depleting so I suggested that she would need to come in to hospital for it to be replaced. The fear in her face and the level of anxiety raised at this suggestion were palpable. It triggered memories of the situation with Janice. I immediately tried to understand her fear and asked her to describe what would be so difficult about coming in. Deep down I thought I knew that she was going to say that the environment restricted her and made her more dependent (Davis & Marsden 2001). This was true: she did start by saying that she would not now, 5 years on from her last admission, be able to use a call bell to attract the nurses. I answered, 'We could look at where to position you on the ward, i.e. to be near the nurses' desk, and I will see if there's any way we could set up a nurse call that you could switch on with your head.'

Still Ann's fear persisted. She is an overweight lady with unpredictable movements and would require careful movement and handling to ensure the safety of all involved. At home her husband lifts her. I thought again that I knew what she was worrying about, the fact that a hoist would need to be used. I asked her and she said, 'Oh no, I know that they will need to hoist me.' She went on, 'I am afraid of the nights the most.' I asked why.

'Normally I have to get up once a night to pass urine,' she explained.

'That would be OK, the nurse would not mind doing that,' I replied.

Ann looked unconvinced. I picked up this cue and said, 'You still look concerned.'

She replied, 'Well yes, because often in the night I need to be moved – you know – every two to three hours.'

I again stated, *'That would be all right, the nurses would be keen to help you with this.'*

Ann then started to talk about how she had never had a pressure sore and she didn't want to get one. I said, *'We'll try to prevent that at all costs.'*

Again there is evidence of glib reassurance (as indicated by italics). By being more mindful, following my experience with Janice, of the fear of coming into hospital, I thought that at several stages I could predict the cause of her anxiety. These views had been influenced by reading related literature (Swain *et al.* 1993; French 1994; Davis & Marsden 2001) and listening to people with disabilities, in particular concerning the difficulties they have in maintaining methods for how they wish to be moved within the current legislation that promotes a no-lift policy for health care workers (Health and Safety Executive 2002). However, despite these previous influences, I really needed to listen and explore what her unique concerns were rather than jumping to conclusions.

Still Ann looked anxious. 'It's something else, isn't it?' I asked. She replied, 'It's getting out in the night to use the toilet, I am so afraid they will say I will have to have a catheter. It's the one thing that I have held on to in all of this, my bladder control, and the last thing my husband and I want is a catheter.'

I said 'I can feel your concern,' and went on to say that if she did not want a catheter she would not have to have one. I felt I really needed to place emphasis on this and concluded by saying that she would not be forced to have one. 'Forced' was quite a strong word to use, but the situation seemed to need it. Finally Ann appeared to start to relax.

CJ asked if it was strong language. I reflected that after so much 'glib reassurance' I felt the need to be more forceful and to use this language to place emphasis on the fact that I was listening and would support her. I was also influenced by my own disappointment that she seemed so disempowered and that just by coming into hospital she felt she would be forced to have an intervention that she did not want. I asked Ann why she thought that might happen, and she recounted how in a previous admission an indwelling catheter had been suggested. This fear was not, then, imagined but a learnt fear from previous experiences. Thinking again from the ward nurse's perspective, I can see how a difficult night toilet transfer could trigger a nurse to wonder how her husband manages, leading to a suggestion of a catheter as a management option.

I stated that I could act as a link between her and the nurses, and that, if things weren't working out, she could tell me and we would try to sort things out together. I closed this discussion by asking her to go home and to brainstorm all the issues she was concerned about and I would ring her the next week to discuss how we could manage them when she came in. She seemed relatively calm when she left the clinic.

In a recent study (Kralik 2002, p. 151), women with chronic illness described different transitions in their lives as they strived to incorporate illness. A quest for ordinariness was interpreted from the women's stories. Ordinariness was described as:

> reconstructing life with illness [which] entailed trying to find a place for illness to fit into their lives. They achieved this by taking calculated risks, surrendering security, making choices and forcing the boundaries that illness had imposed on their lives.

Reading this made me reflect on how Ann and her husband strove for ordinariness in their lives; in particular how they carried out transfers and wanted to maintain their method of managing her bladder. This quest for ordinariness was also evident with Janice, for instance when her husband requested that she sat out for 3–4 hours each day and that her bowel regime be followed.

Without reflecting on my experience with Janice, I do not think I would have pursued Ann's fears as much as I did. I would have relied on what I thought her concerns were rather than uncovering what was fuelling her real reluctance to be admitted. I was telephoned by a hospital manager at 1700 on the following Friday and asked if it would be appropriate to call Ann and ask her to come in at short notice over the weekend. Although her pump needed replacing and could effectively stop at any time, I didn't think she was psychologically ready to come in. However, in the NHS, restricted resources mean that available beds are scarce. Turning down a bed is uncommon, and despite my explanations this was met with slight disbelief from the hospital manager who thought she was doing Ann a favour. She pointed out that not taking this opportunity could delay her admission. Despite this I stated that, although she needed to come in, if we rushed the admission I thought that it would make the duration of her stay longer. *I had no real evidence for this*, but did think this was probably a key card to play with the manager. It turned out to be so and I managed to plan her admission for 6 days later which would give me a chance to further prepare Ann and arrange her surgery to occur quickly after admission so as to ensure as short an admission as possible.

CJ challenged why I thought I didn't have any evidence. Was I looking for empirical evidence? Was my knowledge of knowing the person not good enough? Indeed, it had given me the confidence not only to refuse the bed but also to negotiate an action plan for 6 days later, which was not normal practice. This plan was important as it gave me courage to prioritise Ann's anxiety management above the risk of her mechanical treatment failing whilst knowing that, if things did start to physically go wrong, we had a relatively short time before being able to admit her.

The following week I telephoned Ann. She had no new issues, so we discussed how together we could best manage her admission. I then told her that we were planning to admit her three days later. Her first words were 'That's good, let's get it over with.' Then she started to panic but I reiterated what we had talked about and she ended the conversation by listing what she needed to do.

I liaised with the nursing team and all went to plan. Ann came in on the Thursday, her needs were met overnight, a urinary catheter was not suggested, her pump was replaced on the Friday and she was discharged the following Monday. I asked her if there was anything else we could have done to make her stay easier. She thought long and hard, and stated: 'There really was nothing more you or the hospital could have done. Everything went so smoothly; the rest had to come from me.' I asked her what she meant and she replied that she had to prepare herself for the fact that things would not be the same as at home. She had to make adaptations to ease her needs such as changing her sleeping position. She stated: 'I know nobody else can position me as comfortably, quickly and easily as my husband. I changed my sleep position so as someone didn't have to try.'

To me this really demonstrates the power of working with people and teamwork. Effective health care has to occur in partnership with all those involved. Each person has a unique role and is interdependent on others to achieve the overall aim, which in this case was an effective admission. I fed Ann's comments back to the team including the hospital manager who had helped me to arrange the admission. They agreed it had been very successful.

CJ stated that this admission seemed like a triumph as it all went so smoothly, a key goal for any organisation. To some extent this was true, but I felt there was probably more that could be routinely done to effectively manage the unique needs of individuals with chronic illness coming into hospital."

Janice and Ann, session 19, 29 November 2002

On further reflection on Janice and Ann's care, I mused as to whether nurses only pay lip service to individualised care. Or is it just asking too much of nurses to care in this way within the current resources available? I also need to take into account that increasingly nurses are coming from different countries and cultures, with widely different nursing experiences and training. At times it is hard for them to grasp the nuances of the UK acute model of care. I then challenge that norm and ask them to look at care in a different way. To promote working in partnership with people and to ease their transition into and out of hospital, I feel I need to improve my communication with the ward nursing staff. This reflection highlights the recurring theme of where I should position myself in order to promote effective working between people with disabilities, the nurses, other professionals and myself.

In response I have collaborated with the ward nurses and the pain management department nurses. We have developed standardised care plans or protocols for the technical aspects of the treatments which enable safe practice to continue with the treatments although, as I have revealed, it does not ensure the associated nursing care. Now I must address the *holistic* aspects of someone's care and needs. Do I need to do a written pre-assessment outlining their needs? Would individual nurses read it? In the past I have handed over key information verbally to the nurses, and with this information and their initial assessment they have planned care. Is this the most effective way to achieve effective care and develop nursing skills? CJ felt that completing an assessment form pre-admission would be a useful way of improving communication. I wasn't sure. I felt that the nurses would not then do their own assessment and would just adopt mine, limiting not only the gathering of further information but also the development of their assessment skills. This I felt might de-skill them. CJ challenged my views: What does it mean to de-skill someone? Why am I there? Was it to improve patient care?

There is a danger that specialist nurses may prevent other staff from gaining knowledge and experience, but to prevent this their role must focus on improving the skills of others (Humphries 1999). Perhaps, as I stated earlier, I should explore doing a joint assessment with the ward nurses, influencing care whilst also being a role model and keeping the person central to the assessment.

I wondered whether I could empower the patient by completing the form with them and giving it to them to bring on admission as well as giving a copy to the ward team. CJ challenged whether these patients are too vulnerable and said that I would need to give it to the nursing team. I still felt sceptical. Janice had come into a ward with a clearly written care plan from the community team but the ward nurses had failed to follow it despite continual prompting from me. Although there is evidence in the literature that community plans do work (Davis & Marsden 2001), in my experience and in this case they did not. This led us to discuss whether perhaps a more general teaching approach to the ward nursing teams was required, in order to explore the issues for people with chronic illness coming into an acute hospital setting before initiating other changes.

Teaching session (session 21, 16 April 2003)

I facilitated a teaching session with one of the neurology ward sisters with the aim of exploring tensions between acute and chronic illness models of care in neurology. As nurses from different areas, including critical care and neurosurgery, attended, I wondered if this would impact on the session. However, as it proceeded, experiences seemed similar. Participants were very animated, and keen to participate and express their views. When I asked how they felt when a person with chronic illness and complex needs was to be admitted, they groaned and said they wondered how it would impact on their workload. They talked of 'tricks', i.e. saying to admissions they would accept them but not until later when their workload was quieter. Some explained that although this often delayed the person arriving on their shift, it enabled work to be completed and planning to occur so that the admitting nurse would have time to devote to completing an appropriate assessment, identifying needs and planning care soon after the person arrived.

One nurse was very insightful about the pressures facing people with chronic illness. She used an example from her practice, which clearly demonstrated skill at negotiation. A patient wanted to use the commode but didn't want to be hoisted. It was not safe to move or transfer him any other way. The nurse explained this to him and gave him the options of hoisting or using a bedpan. When he couldn't decide she didn't pressurise him, giving him time to consider the options; he chose the bedpan. This gave him choice and an element of control. Although it could be argued he was pressurised by needing to go to the toilet, she felt from that moment of negotiation they worked well together during his admission. I used this example (rather than the one I had) to illustrate differences in power between health care professions and patients, and how, if we work to balance power, it can impact positively on current and subsequent interactions. Being flexible and using this experience I think enhanced the messages that I was trying to get across. The nurses seemed to be able to relate to their colleague's story. Perhaps if I had used one of my experiences it might have appeared remote from their practice and so the messages might not have been as effectively understood.

I felt energised after the session, especially as this group of nurses were able to articulate how difficult it can be for people with chronic illness coming into an acute environment and the importance of listening to their families and carers about their care needs. I wondered how, or if, the session would impact on their practice. When I asked this of the group at the end of the session, a few replied, and others nodded with agreement, that as a result of the session they would think the next time they nursed an individual with chronic illness about the issues that had been raised. However, a nagging doubt haunted me: would they? It would be difficult to fully assess this. I will need to continue to reflect on these issues to see if other strategies relating to documentation may be useful.

CJ felt the teaching was an important experience as a marker of expanding my CNS teaching role in taking direct and valid action to influence care.

Evidence of reflexivity

Both experiences help me to focus on an important aspect of my role and development of skills: easing the path for people with complex disabilities to come in, through and out of hospital. Predominantly this was triggered by recognising that people with complex needs fear being admitted to hospital. When nursing people I try to identify how they maintain the ordinariness of their lives (Kralik 2002), and how this involves their main carer or family member. Coming into hospital, a large disruption for most people can become an even bigger deal if you have complex needs. Often the impact is as big for the carer who may take the lead in trying to negotiate care rather than doing it.

Precarious harmony

Reflecting in my journal on how I perceived that people with disabilities cope on a daily basis I wrote:

> "It feels as if when at home they live in a precarious harmony teetering on a precipice of coping or not with their daily needs. Yet through a detailed routine, which varies very little, this precarious harmony establishes a lifestyle that works for the individual and their family. Although what is particularly striking is that even the smallest variation in routine can lead to a breakdown in their equilibrium which can take months to restore to their precarious harmony."

Such small variations in routine can occur in hospital and be an unwanted legacy long after discharge home. In trying to support people I find I am living out a tension moving between advocacy and paternalism. It is hard to enable disabled people to be in control within acute care. To try to enable this I adopt a parental role to prop the individuals up during an admission. It is a crucial role. If I did not do this, they would have less chance to assert their perspective and try to preserve their precarious harmony for discharge. I act as a link between the individual and the hospital system. I am continually trying to limit the time it may take them to re-establish their equilibrium or precarious harmony once they get home.

When looking at hospital admissions for people with complex needs, I am now more mindful of listening to their stories, especially in respect of how they manage their level of disability. I am certainly more mindful of the tensions between chronic and acute illness models and in positioning myself with ward nurses in ways that promote the best interests of patients such as Janice and Ann and their families. Listening to and appreciating the patient's perspectives, and on that basis negotiating an acceptable pattern of care, are fundamental. Yet I do not have authority over the ward nurses, and so I must be in a position to ensure that such negotiated patterns are realistic – hence the collaboration with ward staff as achieved with Ann's care. I now more actively share information and have started to question how I can be more of an ongoing support to enable them to develop skills to practise effectively with people who have complex disabilities.

I remember how in the past I would use the admissions of people with chronic illness as an ideal opportunity to carry out an extensive multidisciplinary assessment, looking at lots of issues with the individual and with other disciplines and seeing what we could suggest to help. Crucial steps missing included valuing the patient's or family's knowledge, and whether they wanted this level of intervention. Further, this approach implies a level of arrogance that we in a hospital setting may have more knowledge than our community colleagues, a theme I have gone on to explore with a group of specialist nurses using experiences from this research (Jarrett 2003). A conclusion is that health care professionals across primary and secondary care need to work more closely together, respecting each other's knowledge and skills, and keeping the needs of the individual as they perceive them as the focus of their work.

Glib reassurance

The way I reassure patients is revealed as significant within the pattern of relationship between the patient and myself. In an early draft for this chapter I wrote:

> "I used glib reassurance with both couples as a way of managing their anxiety. Perhaps a certain level is needed to enable progression in the discussion and deeper questioning to identify the real issues. Perhaps the individual statements do not reassure as certainly Ann continued to look anxious. However, collectively the statements of glib reassurance may demonstrate that someone is listening and available to help problem solve issues, enabling a safe environment for the real issue of concern to be disclosed."

CJ challenged this passage and stated that nurses reassure to relieve their own anxieties not those of others. He said that, contrary to what I stated, reassurance closes down discussions; it doesn't move them on to allow deeper feelings to be shared. These observations are backed up in the literature. Reassurance has been defined as an attempt to communicate with people who are anxious, worried or distressed with the intention of inducing them to predict that they are safe or safer than they presently believe or fear (Teasdale

1995). When used it can deny patients the opportunity to express emotions (Hayes & Larson 1963; Balint 1964 cited in Teasdale 1995) or stop the professional from saying the wrong thing (Kirkham 1987, cited in Teasdale 1995) and is usually a matter of the therapist reassuring himself rather than the patient (Sullivan 1954, cited in Teasdale 1995).

I was using reassurance as Teasdale (1995) describes, but I was not aware that I was doing this to stem my own anxieties. I believed I was using it to make them feel safer and to further the conversation, not to stifle it. Rather than stopping myself from saying the wrong thing I was saying something to demonstrate I was listening, trying to plan and problem-solve ways of managing the issues raised. Perhaps, however, how I could use my role to influence the planning and problem solving aspects was not explicit. Instead the body language they saw and the words they heard showed immediate concern but not how I could impact on their actual admission experience. In future, as with Ann, I need to be explicit about how I can support them.

Reassurance can be appropriate to use with people who have a chronic illness when it induces them to maintain hope and confidence in their own abilities (Buchsbaum 1986). I was trying to work with these two couples to convey to them what they knew, and that how they managed their condition was important. But who was it important for: me, the ward staff, the hospital managers? Probably myself: I was trying to ease my own anxieties that although I respect the skills and knowledge of individuals about their disease and management strategies, this may be at odds with how they will be viewed in the acute hospital setting. Reflecting now, both Janice and Ann and their respective families were not new to hospital admissions. They probably thought similarly, that their views would not be respected. Research into relationships between health care providers and people with chronic illness (Thorne & Robinson 1988) describes three ways people can react to health care staff. Initial encounters start with 'naïve trusting' based on the individual's/family's assumption that their experience with illness will be understood and that their personal involvement and knowledge will be acknowledged and valued leading to collaborative goal setting. When this doesn't occur, it leads to 'disenchantment' characterised by dissatisfaction with care, frustration, fear and loss of trust in the health care system. For some these feelings remain. Others have to forge a relationship because something else happens that requires health care intervention. They will either go on to trust individuals known to them or will seek a relationship of 'guarded alliance' where mutual trust is reconstructed and control is shared.

I certainly feel I was working to maintain/reconstruct a guarded alliance, and can now see that the use of glib reassurance could jeopardise this level of trust, pushing my relationship back into the realms of disenchantment. I need to be alert to this emerging thread with subsequent experiences.

Five intervention categories have been described as used by nurses to calm anxious patients: using prediction, giving support, patient control, distraction and direct action (Teasdale 1995). Of these only prediction and giving support were stated as relating to reassurance, both of which I feel were evident in my interaction with Ann. However, I also think our joint planning and negotiation about her admission or the 'direct action' did contribute to easing her anxieties and reassuring her. Similarly, I was trying to give Janice and Ann control by asking about their daily routines, encouraging them to describe what they may need, thus helping us to jointly plan how their routine could fit into that of the hospital. It could be argued that this initially raised their anxieties rather than reassuring them. However, in the longer term this strategy encouraged Ann to reframe the situation and adapt herself psychologically to view the admission in a new, more positive light or (relating to the reassurance definition) to view the admission as safer than she viewed it previously. It was certainly empowering for her in that she changed her night sleeping position.

Loss of control during hospitalisation and gaining back control over one's situation can be a form of reassurance (Fareed 1996). I feel as if I am trying to minimise loss of control for people so as to enable them to have a smooth transition in, through and out of hospital. I am more mindful of my own anxiety and of the need to respond to the patient's or family member's anxiety, which are additional threads to pick up in subsequent experiences.

CJ's reflection

Remember these are Lou's 18th and 19th guided reflection sessions. Put another way, we have been working together for over 18 months. The focus for her reflections is absolutely central to her vision and role in working with chronically ill people who require hospital admission for spasticity treatment. Her reflection reveals how vulnerable and precarious the hospital admission is for patients because nursing staff are locked into a particular view of nursing that fails to listen to people in terms of their needs. The teaching session further revealed a prevailing negative attitude towards such persons – a point that can be substantiated in the chronic illness literature. As a result people like Janice and Ann are likely to suffer more rather than have their suffering eased. Lou positions herself within this dilemma and works to understand and ease suffering. This is the major theme that runs through all her sessions – to create the conditions within practice for her to be available to her patients and their families (see Box 12.1). As Lou highlights, the forces embedded in the care culture constrain her availability and are not so easily shifted even when understood. I use the metaphor of 'chipping away', with perseverance (what I term as reality perspective framing – Johns 2002).

The text also gives insight into the impact of the other 'being available' domains, notably: knowing the person, aesthetic response (the example of reassurance), and knowing and managing herself within a relationship (using reassurance to manage her own anxiety). Lou's concern drives the whole process. At times she has reflected on her despair, and used reflection to pick herself up. Without doubt her narrative reveals the significance of the reflective process to sustain her through understanding, empowerment, action and reflection. Even as we apply the 'being available' template, we are mindful of its 'validity' to mark Lou's reflexive journey of realising her vision (of spasticity nursing) as a lived reality. Her vision is always conscious, rippling through her written word as we seek meaning. It is one thing to hold an idea or concept in the mind, it is quite another to live it meaningfully in practice.

In terms of narrative process, Lou is sophisticated in reflection between sessions, for example in the way she draws the links between Janice and Ann's care. Lou viewed Janice's experience as a negative exemplar. It raised a number of issues that Lou could demonstrate she had responded to in Ann's experience. Between sessions 18 and 19, Lou acted by facilitating a teaching session that enabled a deeper reflection on the developmental themes amplified within the sessions and threading through the unfolding narrative.

The reflexive spiral

For the narrative to be truly reflexive, i.e. to capture the immediacy of the unfolding drama, it is vital that it be written as it unfolds rather than as a retrospective exercise. Within the unfolding it is vital too to capture the guidance process to illuminate the developmental process and as a transparent trail of fusing horizons (Johns 2002). I prefer to structure the narrative through each guided reflection session simply because each session offers a pause to reflect more deeply on situations, and to draw insights to springboard Lou into the mystery of her future practice.

References

Belenky, M., Clinchy, B., Goldberger, N. and Tarule, J. (1986) *Women's Ways of Knowing: The Development of Self, Voice, and Mind*. Basic Books, New York.

Buchsbaum, D.G. (1986) Reassurance reconsidered. *Social Science and Medicine*, **23**(4): 423–7.

Carper, B. (1978) Fundamental patterns of knowing in nursing. *Advances in Nursing Science*, **1**(1): 13–23.

Davis, S. and Marsden, R. (2001) Disabled people in hospital: evaluating the CNS role. *Nursing Standard*, **15**(21): 33–7.

Fareed, A. (1996) The experience of reassurance: patient's perspectives. *Journal of Advanced Nursing*, **23**(2): 272–9.

Fay, B. (1987) *Critical Social Science*. Polity Press, Cambridge.

French, S. (1994) *On Equal Terms. Working with Disabled People*. Butterworth-Heinemann, London.

Harrison, J. (1993) Medical responsibilities to disabled people. In *Disabling Barriers: Enabling Environments* (Swain, J., Finkelstein, V., French, S. & Oliver, M., eds), pp. 211–17. Sage, London.

Health and Safety Executive (2002) *Handling Home Care*. HSE Books, Sudbury.

Humphries, D. (1999) A framework to evaluate the role of nurse specialists. *Professional Nurse*, **6**: 377–9.

Jarrett, L. (2003) Attitudes to long-term care in multiple sclerosis. *Nursing Standard*, **17**(17): 39–43.

Jarrett, L., Leary, S., Porter, B., Richardson, D., Rosso, T., Powell, M. and Thompson, A.J. (2001) Managing spasticity in people with multiple sclerosis. A goal orientated approach to intrathecal baclofen therapy. *International Journal of MS Care*, **3**(2): 10–21.

Jarrett, L., Nandi, P. and Thompson, A.J. (2002) Managing severe lower limb spasticity in multiple sclerosis: does intrathecal phenol have a role? *Journal of Neurology, Neurosurgery and Psychiatry*, **73**: 705–9.

Johns, C. (1995) Framing learning through reflection within Carper's fundamental ways of knowing. *Journal of Advanced Nursing*, **22**: 226–34.

Johns, C. (2002) *Guided Reflection: Advancing Practice*. Blackwell Science, Oxford.

Johns, C. (2004a) *Becoming a Reflective Practitioner*, 2nd edn. Blackwell Publishing, Oxford.

Johns, C. (2004b) *Being Mindful, Easing Suffering: Reflections on Palliative Care*. Jessica Kingsley, London.

Johns, C. and Freshwater, D. (1998) Preface to *Transforming Nursing through Reflective Practice*. Blackwell Science, Oxford.

Jones, B. and Jones, G. (1996) *Earth Dance Drum*. Commune-a-Key Publishing, Salt Lake City.

Kieffer, C. (1984) Citizen empowerment: a developmental perspective. *Prevention in Human Services*, **84**(3): 9–36.

Kralik, D. (2002) Women's experiences of 'being diagnosed' with a long-term illness. *Journal of Advanced Nursing*, **33**(5): 594–602.

Pirsig, R. (1974) *Zen and the Art of Motorcycle Maintenance*. Vintage, London.

Roberts, S. (2000) Development of a positive professional identity: liberating oneself from the oppressor within. *Advances in Nursing Science*, **22**(4): 71–82.

Sullivan, H.S. (1954) *The Psychiatric Interview*. Tavistock, London.

Swain, J., Finkelstein, V., French, S. and Oliver, M. (1993) *Disabling Barriers: Enabling Environments*. Sage Publications, London.

Teasdale, K. (1995) Theoretical and practical considerations on the use of reassurance in the nursing management of anxious patients. *Journal of Advanced Nursing*, **22**(1): 79–86.

Thorne, S.E. and Robinson, C.A. (1988) Health care relationships: the chronic illness perspective. *Research in Nursing and Health*, **11**: 293–300.

Waterlow, J. (1985) A risk assessment card. *Nursing Times*, **81**(49): 51–5.

Index